From the Chief Medical Officer

The impact of climate and climate change on health is a subject I have mentioned before in these editorials. My thoughts returned to this matter during April of this year - a time when many areas of the United Kingdom (UK) were affected by snow storms, torrential rain and flooding. It was at this time I came across a publication from the University of East Anglia entitled *Economic impacts of the hot summer and unusually warm year of 1995*[1]. This document reviews a wide range of environmental issues including impacts on: forestry; agriculture; water; energy; manufacturing; construction; transport and tourism. There is also a health section covering heat wave deaths and winter deaths, and the issue of food poisoning. It is a fascinating read and shows just how much the weather can influence our culture, environment and health.

Infection and the possible risk to public health is another issue which has featured in these editorials. I am therefore pleased to be able to draw attention to a new journal which was launched recently, *Communicable Disease and Public Health*. Published by the Public Health Laboratory Service in association with the Scottish Centre for Infection and Environmental Health, it contains reviews, original articles and short reports. This will be an important journal for anyone interested in infection and its impact on public health.

Research and development (R&D) have a high priority within the health service, and the recent publication of a report of a National Working Group on R&D in primary care[2] is a good example of how the research culture is increasingly being embedded in the health service as a whole. It covers a wide range of issues and makes a number of important recommendations in relation to funding, co-ordination with other research interests such as the Medical Research Council (MRC), the importance of developing regional primary care networks and the provision of training opportunities. At the same time, the MRC has published its most recent booklet on *Guidelines for good clinical practice in clinical trials*[3]. The guidelines relate directly to the 13 principles laid down by the International Conference on Harmonisation Tripartite Guideline for Good Clinical Practice which were agreed in Europe in 1996 and should be read by all those involved in clinical trial research.

Genetics and molecular biology have an increasing role to play in the management of patients, and in developments to improve health. The ability to test for genetic disease, for example, provides the possibility of prevention or early diagnosis. However, there are a variety of ethical issues which need to be considered, and it was for this reason that the Advisory Committee on Genetic Testing was set up. The Committee published its first annual report in March[4], in which it describes the Code of Practice and guidance on human genetic testing services which are supplied directly to the public. It is also considering genetic testing for late-onset disorders and other developments. In such a rapidly developing area it is important to have clear guidelines, and that such guidelines are widely disseminated and considered by the public at large.

The power of computers in assisting clinical research and the management of patients is now well recognised. Developments on the technical side have provided solutions to many different issues, but some fundamental problems remain. With this in mind, the Clinical Systems Group, which I chair jointly with the Chief Nursing Officer, was set up to look at some of the broad issues related to information technology (IT). As part of this process three reviews were commissioned, and these have been published in a document entitled *Improving clinical communications*[5]. The first review concerns health data and how it is transferred between different professionals involved in the management of individual patients. This fascinating study shows how far we still have to go in sharing and using information. The other reviews cover patient and professional views on the communication of clinical information between professionals, and the importance of education and cultural change in the use of information. Taken together, these three reviews provide valuable information from which lessons can be learned about how we communicate and how that communication could be improved.

Earlier this year two important documents covering health services for people with learning disabilities were published. These were prepared by the NHS Executive after extensive consultation with professionals, service users and carers. Good practice guidance is contained in *Signposts for success in commissioning and providing health services for people with learning disabilities*[6], which draws attention to the importance of all health services responding appropriately to people with special needs. This is in line with the themes of social inclusion and of agencies working together effectively, described in *Our Healthier Nation*[7] and *The new NHS: modern, dependable*[8]. It is important that we all recognise that people with special needs expect and deserve to be treated equally and with respect. *The healthy way*[9] is an interactive guide for people with learning disabilities, available with an audiotape version and poster game. It encourages people to think about the health service, and to identify the help that they need and how to seek it.

As usual I have been out and about over the last few months. I visited the North West recently, where I was able to see an interesting safety initiative in Burnley, a fascinating development in Blackburn related to ethnic minority health, and a well-supported community food co-operative in Chorley. In 1995, Lancashire County Council and Burnley Borough Council, working with Lancashire Constabulary, East Lancashire Health Authority and Burnley Health Care NHS Trust, submitted a bid for the Government's £5 million Safe Town Demonstration Project. This resulted in Burnley being selected as one of two runners-up and, in view of the high quality of the bid, an additional £200,000 in Supplementary Credit Approvals were made available in Lancashire for 1996/97. This grant was spent on a package of measures in Burnley known as the 'Southwest Burnley Safety Initiative'. The primary purpose of this initiative was to reduce the incidence and severity of road accidents in the area, especially those involving children and other pedestrians. Additionally, the residential environment was to be improved thereby encouraging children (with their parents) to walk to and from school. The scheme comprised traffic calming measures and the 'Safer routes to school' campaign. These routes were marked on the footway by coloured stencils of 'footprints' and were publicised by leaflets to households and a work-pack for use in schools. An initial evaluation of the initiative suggests that the number of accidents has fallen by 36%. However, no large change in the number of children walking to school has been seen, and parental comments show that further work is necessary to reduce the risk to children and parents' perceptions of these risks.

Partnership between the community, health services and local authority was evident in the development of a food co-operative at the Clayton Brook Village Hall in Chorley. Local residents had expressed their concern about the availability of cheap fresh fruit and vegetables in the locality - a somewhat isolated estate on the outskirts of Chorley. With the support of the health authority and local authority, volunteers from the community have formed a planning group to organise a food co-operative. This operates once a week from the Village Hall and has a growing and enthusiastic membership.

The Brookhouse ward in Blackburn is the most deprived part of that town (on the basis of Jarman scores) and one of the most deprived in the country. Eighty per cent of the population in the ward are from ethnic minority groups. Based around Bangor Street, in the centre of the ward, a 'Bangor Street Project' aims to improve local facilities, and to address the health, social and educational needs of the population. It is a multi-agency initiative supported by local community action. Following on from the 'City Challenge' programme which started in 1991, the area now has many new facilities such as: a social services day centre with attached nursery; a community health and medical centre; a day centre for elderly Asian residents managed by Age Concern; a youth and community centre; and various linking services. Specific health needs which are being addressed include: child nutrition; diabetes mellitus; ischaemic heart disease risk-factors; family planning; and mental health. Above all there is a strong desire expressed by the community for a better understanding of health and how to make the best of health services. The active partnership between the health services and the local community is a key factor in taking this initiative forward, and it is most welcome development.

Kenneth C. Calman

References

1. Palutikof JP, Subak S, Agnew MD. *Economic impacts of the hot summer and unusually warm year of 1995.* Norwich: University of East Anglia, 1997.
2. *Research and development in primary care: National Working Group report.* Department of Health, 1998.
3. Medical Research Council. *Guidelines for good clinical practice in clinical trials.* London: Medical Research Council, 1998.
4. Advisory Committee on Genetic Testing. *Advisory Committee on Genetic Testing: first annual report July 1996-December 1997.* London: Department of Health, 1998.
5. Clinical Systems Group, Department of Health NHS Executive. *Improving clinical communications.* Leeds: Department of Health, 1998.
6. Department of Health. *Signposts for success in commissioning and providing health services for people with learning disabilities.* London: Department of Health, 1998.
7. Department of Health. *Our Healthier Nation: a contract for health.* London: Stationery Office, 1998 (Cm. 3852).
8. Department of Health. *The new NHS: modern, dependable.* London: Stationery Office, 1997 (Cm. 3807).
9. Department of Health. *The healthy way.* London: Department of Health, 1998.

Reviews

The origin and first half of the National Health Service

George Godber

Formerly Chief Medical Officer, England.

Correspondent: Sir George Godber, c/o Health Trends, Room 100, Eileen House, 80-94 Newington Causeway, London SE1 6EF.

Health Trends 1998; **30**: 3-4

Before 1948, we had pieces of a health service, some provided by voluntary bodies, some by local authorities, either under public health or public assistance powers but without co-ordination. Sometimes there was overlap, sometimes even hostility and there were inevitable gaps which the poorest groups could ill afford to fill. In World War II, services for 'casualties' were organised by the Health Departments and a 'casualty' could be anything from someone with a major injury in an air-raid to a child evacuee in a provincial town who needed a tonsillectomy. We all knew that a coherently organised service for everyone must come and this was confirmed by Beveridge and by the guidance given to the regional teams of surveyors who reviewed all our hospitals under the aegis of the Health Departments and the Nuffield Trust in 1942-44. A White Paper was published in 1944[1] and negotiation began. But real definition only came with Aneurin Bevan's arrival as Minister of Health in 1945, and his affirmation that the proposed National Health Service (NHS) would be for all, free at the time of use, mainly financed from taxation and that the hospitals would be nationalised. The National Health Service Act[2] was passed in mid-1946 and the NHS came into effect on 5 July 1948.

There were three arms to the service - the region/district system of hospitals and specialist services; the primary care services of medicine, dentistry, pharmacy and optometry; and the community support and public health services of counties and county boroughs. It looked complicated, but at least the primary care and public health services were the direct successors of existing bodies. It was only the regional organisation of hospitals and the district management that were entirely new. Even so, we had much to learn and do before the appointed day and nearly failed to get the medical profession's agreement. On 5 July 1948 the NHS did work; that happened because the health professions simply cared for people as they had before. It was only the source of payment and the office work that changed.

Fifty years ago we were at the beginning of a period of continuously accelerating change in the sciences related to health. None of us could be aware of the changes that would be needed, even if we could develop the NHS to meet the needs we did then understand; and there was much needed to do that. The writer was involved for the first twenty-five years, twenty-three of them as Deputy or Chief Medical Officer, and this note can only mention a few major developments. Wilson Jameson was Nye Bevan's first Chief Medical Officer, and John Charles followed him for the ten years to 1960.

The hospital and specialist services were regrouped in every district within each of the fourteen, later fifteen, regions of England and Wales. Medical staff were graded by professional committees set up by the Regional Boards and the number of consultants roughly doubled in the first 25 years. That increase was mainly in specialties other than general medicine and surgery, which had been dominant, and we ended with a complete pattern of the specialties in every region, and access to them from every district. Where we failed was in securing a proper balance of junior and senior staff, so that young specialists were kept back too long as registrars and senior registrars. But the outcome in service to patients was shown in greatly increased turnover, steady reduction in mortality - for instance related to anaesthesia - and continuously extending capacity for intervention. It was not enough, so that waiting time for admission grew almost as a system of clandestine rationing, but the cost was thereby contained.

The pace of scientific change in medicine constantly increased in diagnosis, in therapy and in prevention. We began to undertake close review of outcome as in the Confidential Enquiry into Maternal Deaths, the Faculty of Anaesthetists' study of deaths related to anaesthesia, the National Birthday Trust's study of neonatal deaths and the Hospital Inpatient Enquiry, and various studies of short-stay surgery; but these were only scratching the surface. Clinical work was not yet organised for continuous review. Nevertheless, there was continuous dialogue with the medical and nursing professions through quarterly meetings with the Joint Consultants Committee and such smaller groups as the Cogwheel Working Party, and through the Standing Medical, Nursing and Maternity Committees of the Central Health Services Council. Because those groups did not deal with remuneration it was possible for both sides to use them as alliances, argumentative as they rightly were.

The largest component of the NHS was, and is, primary care. It carried the heaviest part of the extra load in 1948, despite being mainly composed of small general medical practices and separate nursing services. General medical practice was unfairly treated in the application of the Spens recommendations on pay and this was rectified four years later by the Dackwerts inquiry. The extra money then available helped a radical restructuring process facilitating group practice to which the general practitioners (GPs) themselves contributed substantially. This still left great anomalies which were eventually corrected by a Charter negotiated in 1966. From that has developed the present system of primary care, mainly in groups including nurses. The establishment of the Royal College of General Practitioners in the early 1950s was one of the major contributions to NHS development, and it has raised the standing and improved the training and content of this largest section of the medical profession, flanked by representation of its interests by the General Medical Services Committee of the British Medical Association.

Given by these two processes parallel organisations of general and specialist medicine, there remained the obvious need each had of the other. A conference on postgraduate education organised by the Nuffield Trust in late 1961 set out to develop from pioneer work at Exeter and Stoke a pattern of postgraduate centres in all hospital groups so that practising doctors in all fields would have the opportunity of continued learning. The other health professions commonly joined in this process, but this note can hardly encompass an account of the parallel changes in nursing, dentistry, pharmacy and optometry. NHS funds for such work were available from 1964. This was, perhaps, the most important single forward step in the first half of the NHS, and the professions initiated and supported it.

The third arm in 1948 included the traditional preventive work of public health, but also considerably extended community services provided by local health authorities in respect of nursing, social support and the rapidly developing preventive work of immunisation against communicable diseases. This early work in health promotion within the NHS is too little recognised. Vaccination against smallpox was long established. Immunisation against diphtheria was already well under way and tetanus, whooping cough, poliomyelitis, measles and rubella were soon to follow. Tuberculosis was about to be greatly reduced by effective drugs, backed up by BCG vaccination. The

mortality and morbidity from all these diseases was reduced by some 90% and the number of days of hospital care by even more. This saving made possible a great increase in hospital care for other diseases in the early years, for which otherwise both funds and beds would have been insufficient. The possibility of preventing non-infectious disease came forward in other ways. Hill and Doll's demonstration of the link between smoking and lung cancer[3] and all the later work which has shown its far wider damaging effects failed to produce comparable preventive action.

The report of the RCP Committee on Smoking and Health in 1962 had world wide acclaim[4]; but 35 years later there has still been too little action against the largest, single avoidable cause of premature death in our society. Action has been taken on other smaller threats such as phenylketonuria and haemolytic disease of the newborn - but they are no threat to wealthy commerce. Now the social factors which influence health are also better understood, but also await remedy.

One cannot think of the first half of the NHS without mentioning other moments of change. Experience of thalidomide led to action to minimise the risks of new and potent drugs. Family planning was profoundly changed by the development of oral contraceptives and then by the Abortion Act 1967[5], which sharply increased the load on hospitals, but also removed one of the main remaining causes of maternal mortality.

Perhaps the most sobering reflection is that after 20 years of the NHS we had only recently begun to analyse the outcome of clinical care with a view to better management, something Donald Acheson had pioneered at Oxford in the mid-1950s. Things have moved on and a great deal has been achieved; much also remains to be done. No doubt the same sentiment will be expressed in 50 years time.

References
1. Ministry of Health, Department of Health for Scotland. *A National Health Service*. London: HMSO, 1994 (Cm. 6502)
2. *National Health Service Act 194*4. London: HMSO, 1944.
3. Doll R, Hill AB. Mortality in relation to smoking: ten years observation of British Doctors. *Br Med J* 1964; **1:** 1399-1410
4. Royal College of Physicians. *Summary of a Report of the Royal College of Physicians of London on Smoking in relation to cancer of the Lung and other Diseases.* London: Pitman, 1962.
5. Ministry of Health. *Abortion Act 1967.* London: HMSO, 1967.

Health and health services: changes over the last seven years

Kenneth Calman

Chief Medical Officer, Department of Health, Richmond House, 79 Whitehall, London SW1A 2NS

Correspondent: Sir Kenneth Calman

Health Trends 1998; **30**: 5-7

This year marks the 50th anniversary of the establishment of the National Health Service (NHS), following the National Health Service Act of 1946[1]. Although some people felt at that time that the organisation fell short of the proposed integrated service needed, the NHS continues to exist and has served the country well.

Whilst other contributed articles in this issue of *Health Trends* encompass different perspectives of changes over these 50 years, I should like to focus on some of the more recent trends which have occurred over the past seven years, during my time as Chief Medical Officer. Even in that short time health has improved in terms of life expectancy, infant mortality and child mortality (see Table 1). Maternal mortality, very low to begin with, has remained about the same.

Not everything however has improved - there is evidence that the gap between the highest and the lowest social classes has increased[2], and a particular concern is the increase in mortality among young men between the ages of 25-29 years since the mid 1980s. Such inequalities in health are high on the priority list at present, and a whole range of different interventions will be required to tackle them.

The health service agenda has been dominated by the development of health strategies, and by changes to the way in which the NHS is managed and organised. The NHS reforms which began in 1989, introduced the purchaser-provider split, fundholding general practices and NHS Trust hospitals. The emphasis was on developing the internal market and in freeing local providers to deliver better quality services. The present Government has announced the intention of reversing some of these changes, in particular to abolish the internal market and to phase out general practice fundholding. The work associated with these changes has dominated the health service over the past ten years as it has been organised and reorganised, and managed and performance managed, in various different ways. In the midst of these management upheavals, professionals at all levels have delivered a high quality service to patients - the main objective of the health service. Increasingly, the public and patients alike are being involved in decision-making, a trend which is to be welcomed, and focus on patients is greater than ever.

In recent years quality of care has been emphasised, with increasing interest in outcomes, effectiveness, audit, guidelines and quality of practice. Much greater emphasis has been placed on reducing the variations in practice and the inequalities in health care which exist[2]. These variations can be observed in almost every aspect of clinical practice, and an active process is required to level out such inequalities. Part of that process was the setting up of the Clinical Outcomes Group, which I chaired jointly with the Chief Nursing Officer. This in itself was an important signal that quality of care was multiprofessional and multidisciplinary. In dealing with such a complex area, the Clinical Outcomes Group was able to give direction to and provide a basis for subsequent developments; notably the establishment of the National Institute for Clinical Excellence and the Commission for Health Improvement.

The development of clinical audit as an integral part of clinical practice was also very much a part of this process. Related to this was the setting up of the Clinical Standards Advisory Group (CSAG), with responsibility for looking at quality of care in a variety of different services. CSAG reports which cover areas

Table 1: *Life expectancy and mortality, England and Wales.*

Year	Life expectancy (in years)		Infant mortality (Rate per 1,000 live births)			Child mortality (Deaths per 1,000 population)						Maternal mortality (Rate per 1,000 total births)
	Males	Females	Persons	Males	Females	Males (age in years)			Females (age in years)			
						1-4	5-9	10-14	1-4	5-9	10-14	
1990	73.2	78.7	7.88	8.9	6.8	0.43	0.20	0.22	0.33	0.14	0.16	0.08
1991	73.4	78.9	7.38	8.3	6.4	0.40	0.21	0.23	0.33	0.16	0.15	0.06
1992	73.8	79.2	6.58	7.3	5.7	0.34	0.18	0.20	0.29	0.14	0.13	0.06
1993	73.8	79.1	6.30	7.0	5.6	0.36	0.16	0.21	0.28	0.12	0.16	0.05
1994	74.4	79.7	6.20	6.9	5.4	0.31	0.16	0.20	0.27	0.11	0.13	0.07
1995	74.3	79.5	6.10	6.9	5.3	0.28	0.16	0.20	0.25	0.12	0.14	0.07
1996	74.6	79.7	6.10	6.9	5.4	0.32	0.13	0.19	0.25	0.11	0.12	0.06

Source: ONS data apart from life expectancy, which has been supplied by the Government Actuary's Department

such as childhood leukaemia, diabetes mellitus, schizophrenia, cleft lip and most recently clinical effectiveness, using stroke as an example - have been instrumental in changing the way in which services are delivered. The reports have encouraged new ways of thinking and have been critical of existing practice. As the CSAG is professionally driven, the impact of the reports has been considerable.

Another way of looking at service delivery was through the development of service frameworks. The first of these related to cancer services in England[3], and set out a non-prescriptive way of improving the way in which cancer services are delivered. Since its publication, there has been considerable change in the configuration of services, and the development of better standards in quality of care. This model has been developed further in terms of paediatric intensive care. Most recently, it has been announced that national service frameworks in cardiovascular disease and mental health will be developed[4] as part of a package of measures to drive up the quality of service to patients. All of these developments have emphasised the importance of a multiprofessional approach to improving care, the role of the patient and the public, and the need for appropriately managed services.

The past seven years have also seen the development of major new health strategies. The first of these, the *Health of the Nation* White Paper[5], was launched in 1992. It set out five key areas - coronary heart disease and stroke, cancer, mental heath, sexual health and HIV/AIDS and accidents, and set targets for the improvement of a range of health indicators. Over a five-year period, it stimulated a huge amount of activity and interest, with a series of projects being developed at local level. Earlier this year, the Government set out proposals for a new health strategy in the Green Paper *Our Healthier Nation*[6]. It proposes four national targets - to reduce deaths from heart disease and stroke, cancer, accidents and suicide and proposes that local areas will be able to set additional local targets to address their own particular priorities. It also emphasises the importance of tackling inequalities in health, and the need to deal with wider health determinants such as employment, education, housing, the environment and poverty.

Preparation of the White Paper on the public health strategy is being informed by responses to the Green Paper and by a project, led by the Chief Medical Officer, to consider how best to strengthen the public health function in England. This has made a number of recommendations, including the need to develop, once again, multiprofessional approaches to improve the health of the public and to encourage all concerned to be involved, by use of a wide range of skills and expertise and by an inquiry into inequalities in health being conducted by my distinguished predecessor as Chief Medical Officer, Sir Donald Acheson.

Communication also has a vital role to play in improving health and health services, not least in the area of public information. The rapidity of modern day media coverage and comment on health issues can easily lead to 'health issues'. To ensure that relevant information reached doctors as quickly as possible, an electronic cascade system (Public Health LINK) was introduced in 1994. It has also been possible to reduce the number of Chief Medical Officer letters by almost 80%, with

important but non-urgent information being sent to doctors in the quarterly *CMO's Update* which summarises issues of importance to doctors, and to a wider group of health professionals. The Department has become more aware of the need for greater understanding of risk, and more effective communication of risk.

Another important part of the development of public health and health services has been a wide ranging consideration of screening for health problems. A National Screening Committee, chaired by the Chief Medical Officer, was set up July 1996. Its primary function is to advise Ministers about the introduction or amendment of national screening programmes. A number of new screening programmes are being considered, for example those relating to colorectal cancer and Down's syndrome and quality control of existing programmes is kept under review.

The possibility of more effective screening has been aided by developments in genetics and molecular biology which have added to our understanding of disease. Of course, such advances raise many technical, ethical and legal issues, which must be discussed fully with public involvement.

The importance of public involvement was also highlighted by a project looking at how emergency services were delivered in a community setting. It became evident that the public needed to know more about the management of acute medical problems, and how best to get information and help. As a result of this, the Government announced the setting up of NHS Direct[7], a telephone advice line which offers help and information directly to the public at any time of the day or night. This service is being piloted currently, but it offers an interesting and exciting way to re-think means of access to health care.

The last few years have seen considerable emphasis placed on catering for those with special health needs. The mentally ill, the very young and the very old may be particularly vulnerable and need special care. The social consequences of providing appropriate care in an appropriate setting have been recognised. In our multicultural society it has also been recognised that people from the black and ethnic minority communities have special health problems. Much greater attention has been paid to these health needs, and to providing a service which reflects those particular needs.

The link between health, health services and social and economic factors has already been mentioned. One example of this is domestic violence, a topic which was identified as a major public health issue in my Annual Report for 1996[8]. Drug abuse is another example of a social issue which affects health, and where the consequences are considerable. The continued co-operation between health services and social services is essential in tackling these problems of the social environment.

When considering the changes which have taken place in the health services, one cannot overlook developments in the primary care setting. General practice in this country has always been of an extremely high standard. Changes in primary health care teams, with a huge increase in practice nursing, the ability of general practitioners to commission secondary care and the coming together of practices in primary care groups have served to emphasise the importance of not only the first contact with the

Table 2: *Topics found in the introduction of the Chief Medical Officer's Annual Report, 1991-96*

1991	Health of black and ethnic minority groups
	Communicable diseases
	Clinical audit and outcomes of health care
	Medical education and manpower
1992	Health of men
	Cigarette smoking in children
	Mentally disordered offenders
	Verocytotoxin - producing *Eschericlia coli*
1993	Health of adolescents
	Asthma
	Genetic factors and disease
	Changing patterns of infectious disease
1994	Health in the workplace
	Equity and quality
	Food poisoning
	Drug and solvent misuse
1995	Risk recommendations and the language of risk
	Mental health
	Antibiotic resistant micro-organisms
	Information technology
	HIV infection and AIDS
1996	The potential for health
	Health of disabled people
	Consent
	Domestic violence
	Air quality and health

patient, but also of a general practitioner service which provides continuity of care to the patients and their families over a long period of time. Certainly the practice with a patient register should remain as the base through which care is given. The primary care team should be recognised as a highly skilled unit which works together and which can also develop together; this can only be to the benefit of patients.

I should like to mention three more factors which have helped to underpin developments of the last seven years. The first of these was the setting up of the NHS Research and Development Strategy. Taken forward initially by Professor Sir Michael Peckham and latterly by Professor John Swales, this has ensured that research is integral to the development of health services. The culture of evaluation, measurement, and of looking at the value of processes and procedures has been an important step forward.

The second development relates to medical education, where have been radical changes in the curricula of almost all medical schools in the United Kingdom. Based on the General Medical Council's document *Tomorrow's Doctors*[9], medical schools are now much more problem based, community focused and able to develop knowledge, skills and attitudes appropriate to caring for patients in the 21st Century. The importance of multidisciplinary team work has, of course, been emphasised. In the area of postgraduate medical training, considerable progress has been made with implementing the reforms of higher specialist training which were approved by the Government in 1993. Over 12,000 trainees in the 53 medical specialties are now following structured training courses encompassing flexibility, choice, competition and regular asessments of progress. In the area of continuing medical education and professional development, there have been significant changes to the way professional bodies consider this issue and, looking ahead, this is likely to be an area of rapid development. All of these changes, once again, are aimed at improving the quality of care provided both to individuals and to the population at large.

The third factor is the incredible expansion in the use of information technology. However, while mentioning the great strides found in this area, one must not forget that certain issues remain to be fully resolved, for example confidentiality and security of information. However, as a tool for improving communication and developing the knowledge-base, the power of information technology has brought considerable benefits.

During my seven years as Chief Medical Officer, my Annual Reports have sought to reflect these changes, and to emphasise each year a series of issues which were thought to be important to bring to the professions' and to the public's attention. A list of these is contained in Table 2. Resulting changes, all directed at improving the health of the people of England, have required a tremendous effort by health professionals, managers, policy-makers and politicians, but it has been a remarkable experience to be part of this process.

References

1. *National Health Service Act 1946.* London: HMSO, 1946.
2. Department of Health. *Variations in health: what can the Department of Health and the NHS do?* London: Department of Health, 1995.
3. Department of Health, Welsh Office. *A policy framework for commissioning cancer services: a report by the Expert Advisory Group on cancer to the Chief Medical Officers of England and Wales: guidance for purchasers and providers of cancer services.* London: Department of Health, 1995.
4. NHS Executive. *National Service Framework.* Wetherby (West Yorkshire): NHS Executive, 1998 (HSG 1998/074).
5. Department of Health. *The Health of the Nation: a strategy for health in England.* London: HMSO, 1992 (Cm. 1986).
6. Department of Health. *Our Healthier Nation: a contract for health.* London: Stationery Office, 1998 (Cm. 3852).
7. Department of Health. *The New NHS: modern and dependable.* London: Stationery Office, 1997 (Cm. 3807).
8. Department of Health. *On the State of the Public Health: the annual report of the Chief Medical Officer of the Department of Health for the year 1996.* London: Stationery Office, 1997; 23-4
9. General Medical Council Education Committee. *Tomorrow's doctors: recommendations on undergraduate medical education.* London: General Medical Council, 1993.

50 years of the National Health Service in Wales

Deirdre Hine

Formerly Chief Medical Officer, Welsh Office, 185 Cathedral Road, Cardiff CF1 9PN.

Correspondent: Dame Deirdre Hine

Health Trends 1998; **30**: 8-9

Even dramatic improvements in the social well-being of the population come, after a time, to be taken for granted. So it has been with the enormous clinical achievements of the National Health Service (NHS) since its establishment 50 years ago. In the late 1980s this familiarity with a free, comprehensive service gave rise not only to increasing demands on the primary and secondary sectors of the NHS for diagnosis and treatment, but also simultaneously, and somewhat paradoxically, to the criticism that what was being provided was a National Sickness rather than a National Health Service.

A striking and influential challenge to that perception occurred in Wales during the period when I was Chief Medical Officer at the Welsh Office (1990-97), by the forging of an explicit link between the activities of the NHS and the overall health of the population. This was achieved following the publication in 1989 of a strategic intent and direction for the NHS in Wales[1] - later, inevitably, known as 'SID'.

Owing much to the World Health Organization's (WHO's) 'Health for All' policy adopted by the 32 member states of the WHO European Region, it predated the *Health of the Nation* initiative[2] in England. Despite the flaws later identified by its critics[3] (too many targets and not enough evidence); the overall goal of the initiative "working with others, the NHS in Wales aims to take the people of Wales into the next century with a level of health on course to compare with the best in Europe" was properly ambitious and theoretically realistic. It was also in many ways ground-breaking.

The documentation to support the SID was produced by the newly formed Health Planning Forum and introduced many in the NHS and the wider public in Wales to the concept of health gain. Gradually the idea that the whole purpose of the NHS was to achieve health gain - defined as adding years to life and life to years - was accepted and even enthusiastically adopted by NHS staff from nursing auxiliaries to consultants. The protocols for investment in health gain (devised as guidance to health authorities on the most effective way to use their resources to achieve health gain by commissioning or purchasing of individual services) introduced and emphasised, by the multidisciplinary manner of their production, a team approach to health care; while the exhortation to "work with others" was an explicit acknowledgement that the NHS was only one of the public services with influence on and responsibility for the health of people in Wales.

The setting of some 200 targets for improvement over the ten health gain areas of maternal and early childhood health, learning disability, injuries, healthy living, mental health, respiratory diseases, cardiovascular diseases, cancers, physical and sensory disability and healthy environments, together with the requirement that each health authority reflect these in a local health strategy to inform their annual purchasing plan, was undoubtedly a somewhat unwieldy and lumbering vehicle - perhaps altogether too much so to achieve early or easily measurable results. However, for the first time the 'Health for All' philosophy became incorporated into a national health service. Indeed the problems of SID were themselves a significant spur to the newly emerging attempts to achieve better measurement and recording of the outcomes of clinical care, thus preparing the ground in Wales for later initiatives on quality of care and clinical effectiveness.

After a period of near eclipse in the middle of the decade - when policy issues were subordinated to the pragmatic needs of meeting health service demand in a timely way, and when strategic planning was out of fashion - the durability of the SID approach is again becoming apparent. The targets have recently been revised[4], reducing them to 15 common to all Welsh health authorities, and the requirement to work towards them reissued. The launch in March of the first of a set of *Health Evidence Bulletins*[5], building through a newly devised rigorous and sophisticated methodology on the foundations of the original protocols, remains faithful to the SID concept.

And what of the impact of all this on the health status of the Welsh population? My annual report for the year 1992[6] detailed dramatic and significant improvement since the report for 1976 - with reductions in death rates and an increase in life expectancy of five years among men and three years for women. There had been a reduction in perinatal and infant mortality rates to less than half their 1976 rates, the death rate from stroke had decreased by almost one quarter, and the uptake of childhood immunisation exceeded 90% in all parts of Wales.

This was no mean achievement for the NHS over a period of 16 years; however later assessments show that we need to improve ever faster if we are to achieve the SID goals. The 1997 annual report records that death rates are still higher and life expectancy shorter in Wales than in most other European countries[7]. Moreover, there are substantial differences in mortality and morbidity between diferent communities in Wales. Death rates from coronary heart disease, lung cancer in men and breast cancer in women are one-and-a-half to two times greater in the Welsh Unitary Authority with the worst health record compared to that with the best. Perhaps a new target should be to eliminate these inequalities and bring the health of the whole of Wales up to the level of the best in Wales by the year 2010.

There is a growing recognition that poor health status is linked to a combination of factors in many of which - relative socio-economic deprivation, unemployment, occupational diseases, poor housing and poor access to healthy lifestyle options, such as diet or facilities for exercise - the NHS can act only as an advocate for change. As the NHS rightly celebrates its undoubted achievements over the past 50 years, we have to acknowledge that much still remains to be done and that only the acceptance of their joint responsibility with the NHS by central Government, local authorities, commerce, industry and the media, and, of course, by the people of Wales themselves - is likely to result in major progress in the new millennium.

References

1. Welsh Health Planning Forum. *Strategic intent and direction for the NHS in Wales.* Cardiff: NHS Directorate in Wales, 1989.
2. Department of Health. *The Health of the Nation: a strategy for health in England.* London: HMSO, 1992 (Cm. 1986)
3. Gabbay J, Stevens A. Towards investing in health gain. *BMJ* 1994; **308**: 1117-8.
4. Welsh Office. *Iechyd Cymru: Welsh health: annual report of the Chief Medical Officer.* Cardiff: Welsh Office, 1997.
5. Nicholas P, Andrews J, Welsh Office. *Maternal and early child health.* Cardiff: University of Wales College, 1998. (Health Evidence Bulletins Wales).
6. Welsh Office. *Iechyd Cymru Welsh health: annual report of the Chief Medical Officer.* Cardiff: Welsh Office, 1993.
7. Welsh Office. *Iechyd Cymru: Welsh Health: annual report of the Chief Medical Officer.* Cardiff: Welsh Office, 1997.

Articles

Health trends over the last 50 years

Sue Kelly[1] Karen Dunnell[2] John Fox[3]

[1]Health Statistician; [2]Director, Demography and Health; [3]Director, Census Population and Health Group; Office for National Statistics, 1 Drummond Gate, London SW1V 2QQ.

Correspondent: Ms Sue Kelly

Health Trends 1998; **30**: 10-5

Summary

- This year we celebrate the 50th anniversary of the NHS, and this article summarises trends in the health of the population of England and Wales over the last 50 years.

- Major improvements in health have included an increase in life expectancy, a fall in infant mortality and a decline in infectious disease. However, we are still faced with many challenges for the future.

Introduction

The National Health Service was established on 5 July 1948, and this year we celebrate its fiftieth anniversary. Before the inception of the NHS, healthcare was a luxury not everyone could afford. The National Health Service Act, which became law in November 1946, promoted 'the establishment in England and Wales of a comprehensive health service designed to secure improvements in the physical and mental health of the people of England and Wales and the prevention, diagnosis and treatment of illness'. This article summarises trends in the health of the population of England and Wales from the late 1940s/early 1950s. It also includes some more recent trends where earlier data were not available. Where possible, the trends are explained in terms of social changes and advances in medical knowledge and practice. All death rates are age-standardised unless otherwise stated, to take into account changes in the age-structure of the population.

Population structure

As background to a presentation of health trends over the last fifty years, it is worth noting the significant changes which have occurred in the population of England and Wales since 1948. These changes relate, in part, to mortality trends (see later). Figure 1 shows the profile of the estimated male and female population in mid-1948 and mid-1996. The total population increased by over a fifth between 1948 and 1996, from 43 million to 52 million. An increase occurred for all ages except the 0-4-year-old age-group, where the population decreased by 9%. In 1948, this age-group accounted for 9% of the total population; by 1996, this proportion had fallen to 6%. The largest increases in the population, between 1948 and 1996, occurred amongst those aged 65 years and over. In particular, the population aged 80 years and over increased by 245%. The number of women in this age-group increased by more than one million, to represent 6% of the female population in 1996. The number of men aged 80 years and over increased by 438,000 to represent 3% of the male population in 1996.

Mortality

Mortality data provide extensive information on long-term trends in health. The actual number of deaths has remained fairly constant since 1948. This is due to a combination of population growth and postponement of death[1]. There has been a marked shift in the distribution of age at death from younger to older age-groups. In 1948, 40% of deaths occurred in those aged under 65 years. By 1996, this proportion had fallen to 17%. The death rate for males fell from 14,051 per million in 1948, to 9,268 per million in 1996, a fall of 34%. The corresponding rates for females were 10,144 and 5,993 deaths per million, a decrease of 41%.

Figure 2 shows the decline in age-specific death rates since 1948. In 1948 mortality rates were higher for males than females in all age-groups, and this remains true today. The highest death rates are in those aged 65 years and over, and these rates declined the least since 1948. Death rates among children aged 1-14 years fell by more than 80% - from 113 per 100,000 in 1948, to 20 per 100,000 in 1996 for boys; and from 94 to 15 per 100,000 for girls. The infant mortality rate (deaths under the age of one year) fell from 39 per thousand live births in 1948 to seven per thousand in 1996 for boys, and from 30 to five deaths per thousand live births for girls.

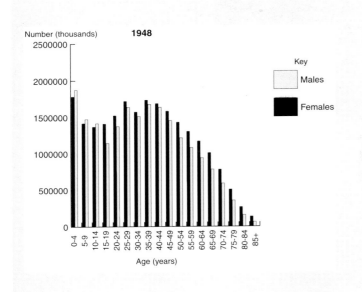

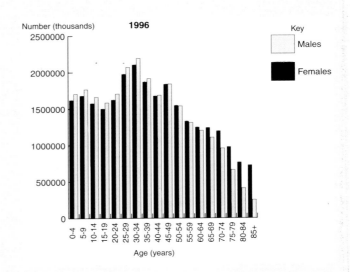

Expectation of life at birth has increased steadily since 1948. For males, it increased from 66.1 years in 1948, to 74.4 in 1995. The corresponding figures for females are 70.5 and 79.6 years. These improvements are due to the declining mortality rates discussed above, which in turn have been influenced by improvements in nutrition, housing, occupational hazards, lifestyle and medical care.

Figure 3 shows differences between 1948 and 1996 in the percentage distribution of the main causes of death. The main changes were a decrease in both the proportion and number of deaths from infectious diseases and genitourinary diseases; and an increase in the proportion and number of deaths from respiratory diseases (particularly among females) and cancer. These increases can partly be explained by the aging population;

it is at older ages that diseases, such as cancer, become manifest. The number of maternal deaths decreased from 809 in 1948, to 41 in 1996. The maternal mortality rate fell from 102 per 100,000 births in 1948, to six per 100,000 births in 1996. The great improvement in the maternal mortality rate from the mid-1930s has been attributed to the introduction of sulphonamide drugs for puerperal sepsis, the availability of penicillin and blood transfusion to women who haemorrhaged[2]. The number of deaths from conditions originating in the perinatal period fell from 12,065 in 1948, to 2,293 in 1985. (A new neonatal death certificate was introduced in 1986, from which it is not possible to assign an underlying cause of death for deaths occurring in the first 28 days of life. The stillbirth rate fell from 23 per thousand total births in 1948, to five per thousand in 1996. These declines were influenced mainly by a range of improvements in diagnosis and care during pregnancy and delivery.

Figure 2: *Age-specific death rates as a percentage of rates in 1948, by sex, England and Wales, 1948-96*

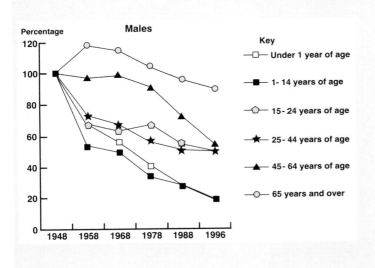

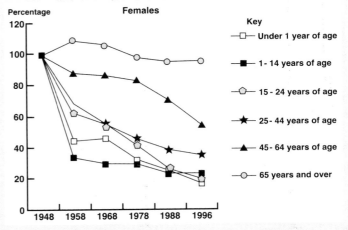

Figure 3: *Mortality: percentage distribution, by cause of death and sex, England and Wales, 1948 and 1996*

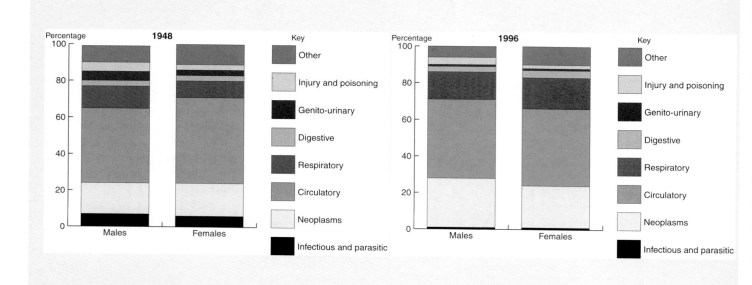

Inequalities

Figure 4 shows a clear social class gradient in infant mortality rates in 1949-50, with the highest rates in the lowest social classes[3]. The gradient is still evident in 1994-95, but is less pronounced[4]. Indeed, in 1994-95 the infant mortality rate was the same for social classes I and II (professional and managerial). The comparison over time was only made for single births inside marriage, as these were the only births for which comparable data were available.

Comparisons of regional patterns in mortality are hindered by the substantial boundary changes that have taken place since 1948. However, even though there was an overall decline in mortality in all regions over this period, the relative pattern of mortality was largely unchanged in 1996 compared with 1948. There persisted a notable regional gradient, with higher mortality rates in the North and North West, and lower rates in the South and East of England.

Specific diseases

Infectious diseases

The fall in mortality rates since 1948, particularly in the youngest age-groups, was due in part to a reduction in the number of deaths from infectious diseases. The introduction of antibiotics resulted in a large decrease in the number of deaths from infectious diseases, from 30,142 in 1948, to 3,636 in 1996. However, mortality rates from infectious diseases only fell until 1983, since when they have been rising. The mortality rate from tuberculosis declined rapidly from the mid-1940s, but the rate of decline has slowed in recent years. The introduction of effective

Figure 4: *Infant mortality rates by father's social class for single births inside marriage, England and Wales, 1949-50 and 1994-95*

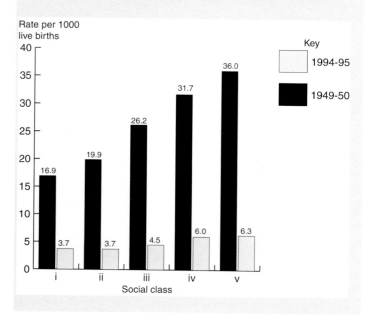

Figure 5: *Notifications of measles, England and Wales, 1940-95*

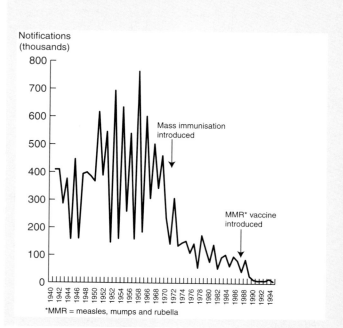

Figure 6: *Days of incapacity per person per year, 1947-51 (England and Wales), and days of restricted activity per person per year, 1975-94 (Great Britain), males and females, aged 15 years and over*

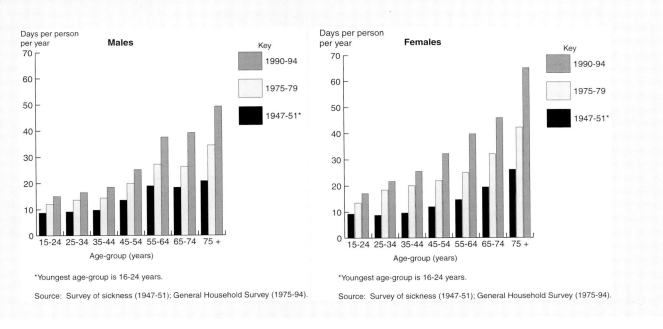

*Youngest age-group is 16-24 years.

Source: Survey of sickness (1947-51); General Household Survey (1975-94).

antibiotics in 1944, 1946 and 1952 had a major impact on death rates. Mass screening for tuberculosis-infected persons took place after the Second World War[5].

Infectious diseases were also a major cause of morbidity in 1948. The number of measles notifications fluctuated around 400,000 between 1948 and 1968. Mass immunisation was then introduced and the number of notifications fell rapidly (Figure 5). Another fall was associated with the introduction of the combined measles, mumps and rubella (MMR) vaccine in 1989. In 1995 there were 7,447 notifications of measles. Trends in notifications of other infectious diseases were similarly affected by the introduction of vaccines.

Cancer
Since the late 1940s cancer mortality rates for males aged 15 years and over have increased by 15%, whilst for women of the same age they have remained fairly stable. However, trends by individual cancer site have followed very different patterns.

Between 1971 (the first year for which national data are available) and 1992, cancer incidence rates increased by 34% in women and 18% in men, although rates continue to be higher amongst men than women. As for cancer mortality, trends in incidence vary by site.

The lung cancer death rate for men increased until the mid-1970s, since when it has been falling. For women, the death rate from lung cancer only started to level off at the start of the 1990s. Trends in age- and sex-specific death rates from lung cancer accord with trends in tobacco consumption, the most important cause of lung cancer (see later). Lung cancer incidence shows a similar trend to that for mortality due to poor survival rates. Despite the falls in incidence, it remains the most common cancer in men.

Unlike the pattern for men, lung cancer incidence showed a substantial increase amongst women, with a rise of 76% in the age-standardised rate (compared to a fall of around 30% in the

rate for men) between 1971 and 1992. The incidence rate among women is slightly lower than the corresponding rate for colorectal cancer, the second most common cancer in women. The incidence of colorectal cancer has remained level over the past decade, so the incidence of lung cancer is likely to exceed it in the next few years, and become the most common cancer in women after breast cancer. Mortality rates from colorectal cancer have fallen for both men and women since the early 1940s.

Since the late 1940s the death rate from prostate cancer increased by 77%. Prostate cancer has shown one of the largest increases in male cancer incidence over the past twenty years, and in 1992 became the second most common cancer in men.

For women, breast cancer death rates increased by 22% between the late 1940s and late 1980s, since when they have started to fall. A substantial rise has occurred in the incidence of breast cancer since 1984, with a steeper increase after 1988, following the introduction of a national screening programme. Whilst the decline in mortality from breast cancer pre-dates screening, the impact of screening is expected to cause a further fall.

Radiotherapy, used alone or in combination with other treatments, has greatly improved the survival chances of cancer patients. Testicular cancer, some childhood malignancies and Hodgkin's disease are particular examples[5]. A substantial decline in mortality from cervical cancer since 1950 has been helped by successful treatment among those diagnosed early enough[5]. Cytotoxic chemotherapy has radically reduced mortality from acute lymphoblastic leukaemia in children. More recently, tamoxifen treatment seems to have increased survival of women with breast cancer[6].

Circulatory disease
The death rate from ischaemic heart disease for males was fairly stable between 1950 and the mid-1970s, since when it has fallen by about 40%, to reach 2,474 per million in 1996. The female

rate has fallen continuously since 1950 to 1,183 per million in 1996. Reduced smoking has contributed to the reduction in mortality from ischaemic heart disease at all ages in the last 20 years[7]. Since about 1970, subcutaneous cardiac pacemakers have played a major role in increasing life expectancy in patients with heart disease[5]. Death rates from cerebrovascular disease have more than halved since 1950, for both males and females.

Injury and poisoning
Deaths from injury and poisoning now account for only 3% of all deaths (4% in 1951). However, accidents, the largest contributor to deaths from injury and poisoning, are the most common cause of death in those aged under 35 years, and therefore contribute significantly to years of working life lost. Most accidents are considered avoidable. Death rates from motor vehicle traffic accidents are three times as high in men as in women. Since the early 1950s, these rates have almost halved for men, whilst among women they have fallen by nearly one-third, both having peaked in the mid-1960s.

Trends in non-fatal accidents are difficult to identify, but the available data sources indicate that during the last 20 years, patterns of consultation and service use have been increasing steadily[8]. The apparent conflict between mortality and morbidity trends may be related to increasing demand for health services from patients with comparatively minor conditions. This may reflect both changing patient expectations and changes in access to services[8].

General morbidity
Data on morbidity are far more limited than those on mortality. For the 1940s the only available source, other than notifications of infectious diseases, is the Survey of Sickness[9]. This monthly survey ran from 1943-52. For later years, morbidity data have been available from the General Household Survey (GHS) since the 1970s, from the four national studies of Morbidity Statistics in General Practice (MSGP), and individual surveys.

Figure 6 compares the number of days of incapacity (days away from work or, for those not usually employed, days confined to the house) per person per year over the period 1947-51 reported in the Survey of Sickness, with the number of days of restricted activity per person per year reported in the GHS for the periods 1975-79 and 1990-94. The two datasets are not totally comparable. In particular, there was a known under-reporting in the Survey of Sickness due to the longer reference period[9] - 2-3 months compared with 2 weeks in the GHS - and people recalling fewer days of illness. The GHS data do show a higher level of restricted activity, and also an increase since 1975. However, data for 1985-89 (not plotted) would suggest that there has been some levelling off in recent years, particularly among women. Levels of incapacity increase with age and, except for men of working age in 1947-51, more days of incapacity have been reported by women.

Over the period 1949-51, the most commonly recorded illnesses were colds, influenza and other respiratory diseases, and rheumatism[9]. These illnesses, together with injuries for people under 65 years-of-age and diseases of the heart and arteries for those over 65 years-of-age, were also the most common reasons for incapacity and medical consultation. In 1991-92 the most common reasons for consultation at general practice were for

diseases of the respiratory system, nervous system and sense organs, and other health-related matters, including family planning, screening and immunisation[10]. Data from the GHS on (limiting) long-standing illness show that, since the mid-1980s, there has been no improvement in general health measured in this way. There is no difference in the proportion of men and women reporting a long-standing illness (about one third), and the difference for limiting long-standing illness is very small.

Health related behaviour
Diet
During the Second World War, rationing and other factors affecting redistribution probably raised nutritional standards for the poor and may also have provided health gains for the wealthy. Energy intakes have decreased steadily since the 1960s in adults and children, which may reflect a more sedentary lifestyle. In the 1950s, affluent households were the greatest consumers of sugars, fats and eggs, but by 1993 their consumption was the lowest. Fat consumption has declined since 1970. Per capita consumption of fresh fruit has increased some 40% since 1950[11]. Despite these dietary changes, the proportion of adults who are obese or overweight has increased. Obesity is a risk factor for coronary heart disease. In 1996, 17% of women and 16% of men aged 16-64 years in England were obese, compared with 8% and 6%, respectively, in 1980 in Great Britain[12,13].

Alcohol
Alcohol consumption in the United Kingdom has risen from 3.7 litres per head per year in 1948, to 7.0 litres per head per year in 1993[14]. Heavy drinking, though undertaken by a small proportion of the population, is associated with morbidity and premature mortality. It is a major factor in liver cirrhosis and liver disease, and also a factor in coronary heart disease and some cancers[15]. The death rate from alcohol-related liver disease in England and Wales has more than doubled since 1950 for both males and females.

Smoking
Tobacco use by men increased up to the end of the Second World War, when it fell slightly before stabilising. After the 1960s it fell substantially. Use by women started much later, and increased rapidly in the Second World War and continued to increase until the 1970s when it began to fall[7]. In 1996 in Great Britain, 29% of males and 28% of females were cigarette smokers, compared with 65% and 41%, respectively, in 1948[16,17]. However, there has been little change amongst the youngest adults over the last ten years, and cigarette smoking among children has increased during the 1990s[18].

Conclusions
There have been major improvements in health over the last 50 years, including an increase in life expectancy of about nine years, a dramatic fall in infant mortality and substantial falls for severe infectious diseases. Medical advances have played their part, increasing our understanding of the causes of illness and disease. Advances in cell and molecular science and bio-engineering may lead to treatments for chronic conditions such as psychiatric illness, multiple sclerosis and arthritis[19].

Future challenges include developing new drugs to overcome strains of bacteria which are resistant to antibiotics. The proportion of older people will continue to rise, especially at very high ages - the challenge is for them to be able to look forward to a healthy old age. Reductions in fatalities from circulatory diseases, cancers, and injury and poisoning offer the greatest scope for increasing life expectancy in the present era[20]. Indeed, the Government's Green Paper *Our Healthier Nation*[21] includes proposed health improvement targets in all these areas. There is also the challenge in tackling increasing rates of smoking in the young, obesity and physical inactivity.

References

1. Charlton J. *Trends in all-cause mortality:* 1841-1994. In: Charlton J, Murphy M (eds). *The health of adult Britain 1841-1994.* London: The Stationery Office, 1997; 17-29 (Vol 1; Decennial Supplement no. 12).

2. Macfarlane A, Mugford M. *Birth counts: statistics of pregnancy and childbirth.* London: HMSO, 1984.

3. Heady JA, Heasman MA. *Social and biological factors in infant mortality.* London: HMSO, 1959 (Studies on Medical and Population Subjects; no. 15).

4. Office for National Statistics. *Mortality statistics: childhood, infant and perinatal, England and Wales.* London: Stationery Office, 1997 (Series DH3; no. 28).

5. Charlton J, Fraser P, Murphy M. *Medical advances and iatrogenesis.* In: Charlton J, Murphy M, eds. *The health of adult Britain 1841-1994.* London: Stationery Office, 1997; 217-229. (Vol 1; Decennial Supplement no. 12).

6. Quinn M, Allen E. Changes in incidence of and mortality from breast cancer in England and Wales since introduction of screening. *BMJ* 1995; **311:** 1391-5.

7. Doll R, Darby S, Whitley E. *Trends in mortality from smoking-related diseases.* In: Charlton J, Murphy M, eds. *The health of adult Britain 1841-1994.* London: The Stationery Office, 1997; 128-155. (Vol 1; Decennial Supplement no. 12).

8. Nicholl J, Coleman P. *Accidents: trends in mortality and morbidity.* In: Charlton J, Murphy M, eds. *The health of adult Britain 1841-1994.* London: Stationery Office, 1997; 158-72. (Vol 2; Decennial Supplement no. 12).

9. Logan WPD, Brooke EM. *The Survey of sickness 1943 to 1952.* London: HMSO, 1957 (Studies on Medical and Population Subjects; no. 12).

10. McCormick A, Fleming D, Charlton J. *Morbidity statistics from general practice: fourth national study, 1991-92.* London: HMSO, 1995. (Series MB5; no. 3).

11. Charlton J, Quaife K. *Trends in diet 1841-1994.* In: Charlton J, Murphy M, eds. *The health of adult Britain 1841-1994.* London: Stationery Office, 1997; 93-113 (Vol 1; Decennial Supplement no. 12).

12. Knight I. *The heights and weights of adults in Great Britain.* London: HMSO, 1984.

13. Prescott-Clarke P, Primatesta P. *Health survey for England 1996: a survey carried out on behalf of the Department of Health.* London: Stationery Office, 1998. (Series HS; no. 6).

14. Brewers' Society. *Statistical handbook: a compilation of drinks industry statistics.* London: Brewers' Society, 1995.

15. Plant MA. Trends in alcohol and illicit drug-related diseases. In: Charlton J, Murphy M, eds. *The health of adult Britain 1841-1994.* London: Stationery Office, 1997; 114-127. (Vol 1; Decennial Supplement no. 12).

16. Wald N, Nicolaides-Bouman A. *UK smoking statistics.* 2nd ed. Oxford: Oxford University Press, 1991.

17. Thomas M, Walker A, Wilmot A, Bennett N. *Living in Britain - results from the 1996 General Household Survey: an interdepartmental survey carried out by ONS between April 1996 and March 1997.* London: Stationery Office, 1998.

18. Jarvis L. *Smoking among secondary school children in 1996: England. An enquiry carried out by Social Survey Division of ONS on behalf of the Department of Health.* London: Stationery Office, 1997.

19. Office for National Statistics. *Britain 1998: an official handbook prepared by the Office for National Statistics.* London: Stationery Office, 1998.

20. Charlton J, Murphy M. *Trends in causes of mortality: 1841-1994 - an overview.* In: Charlton J, Murphy M, eds. *The health of adult Britain 1841-1994.* London: Stationery Office, 1997; 30-57 (Vol 1; Decennial Supplement no. 12).

21. Department of Health. *Our Healthier Nation: a contract for health.* London: Stationery Office, 1998 (Cm. 3852).

The Goodenough Report and medical education in 50 years of the National Health Service

John Biggs

Postgraduate Dean, University of Cambridge and Anglia and Oxford Region, The Clinical School, Addenbrooke's Hospital, Cambridge CB2 4SP.

Correspondent: Dr J Biggs

Health Trends 1998; **30**: 16-9

Summary

- Sir William Goodenough chaired a committee to inquire into medical schools, with particular regard to facilities for clinical teaching and research. The committee was to look at medical education and the organisation of hospital services in London and nationally, and postgraduate medical education. Its 1944 report has influenced policy and practice in medical education in medical schools and hospitals throughout the 50 years of the National Health Service, but the full expectations of Goodenough have still to be achieved.

Introduction

In March 1942, in the depth of war, the British government established a committee to inquire into the organisation of medical schools and the facilities for clinical teaching and research. Particular attention was to be given to medical education in London, the organisation of hospital services nationally, and the arrangements for postgraduate teaching and research. The committee, chaired by Sir William Goodenough, reported in 1944[1]. It believed its recommendations were evolutionary and would have far-reaching results.

The foundations of a national health service had been laid in the Beveridge report of 1942[2] which recommended 'Comprehensive health and rehabilitation services for prevention and cure of disease and restoration for capacity for work, available to all members of the community'. The Goodenough report was a further part of Government planning for post-war and thus provided a major building block for the future health service. Goodenough contended that medical education was an essential part of a comprehensive health service and this paper looks at his committee's report and its recommendations, and their influence upon the National Health Service (NHS) in its first 50 years.

The Committee

The Committee comprised members of great achievement and experience. The chairman, aged 43, was deputy chairman of Barclays Bank, director of Commercial Union Assurance and chairman of numerous boards and committees including the Nuffield Trust for the medical school of Oxford University and the Trustees of Nuffield College, Oxford. Sir John Stopford FRS was Vice-Chancellor and Professor of Experimental Neurology of Manchester University. Professor Thomas Elliott FRS was consultant physician at University College Hospital (UCH) and emeritus professor of medicine at London University. Dr Archibald Gray was consultant dermatologist and dean of the medical school at UCH. Professor James Hendry was Regius professor of midwifery at Glasgow University and medical director of the Royal Maternity and Women's Hospital, Glasgow. Professor A V Hill FRS had won the Nobel Prize for physiology and medicine in 1922 and had honorary doctorates from six international universities: he was a professor of the Royal Society, Member of Parliament for Cambridge University, and a member of the War Cabinet scientific advisory committee. Sir Wilson Jameson, MD, was Chief Medical Officer of the Ministry of Health and the Board of Education, and a member of the Medical Research Council. Professor James Learmonth was professor of surgery at Edinburgh University. Sir Ernest Pooley, barrister at law and clerk to the Drapers' Company was a member of the Senate and Court of the University of London. Dr Janet Vaughan, eminent haematologist, was in charge of blood supply in north-west London; she was later to become Principal of Somerville College, Oxford.

The report

It was said of the Committee that 'few bodies in the history of medicine have had a greater opportunity or more responsibility'[3]. It produced an extraordinary report that addressed all aspects of medical education, the relationships of universities and hospitals, and future needs for a national health service. A major emphasis in Goodenough was on the essential nature of medical education in the nation's hospitals and the point is made again and again: "The interests of both patients and students are served if, in the framing of policy and the conduct of the hospital's affairs, the two functions of a teaching hospital, namely the care of patients and the furtherance of teaching and research, receive equal emphasis, being regarded as complementary and mutually reinforcing"[4].

The Committee's view may have resulted from the shortcomings of the disconnected system of voluntary and municipal hospitals that then existed, or from the exigencies of a system under the strains of war, but the feelings were clearly expressed: "The spirit of education must permeate the whole of the health service, and that service must be so designed and conducted that, among other things, it secures for medical education the necessary staff, accommodation, equipment and facilities. Medical education cannot be regarded as merely incidental to the hospital service"[5]. Rivett[6] claimed that the members of the committee were appointed by Government to reflect its views on medical education, but in any case, its report was accepted by Government and many of its findings were built into the national health service that was to follow. After 50 years of the service it can be asked how far the principles and recommendations of Goodenough have been followed, and the place of medical education in the NHS established.

Undergraduate education

Among many recommendations on the structure and work of medical schools, Goodenough proposed, as the basic unit for undergraduate medical education, a 'medical teaching centre' comprising a university medical school, a teaching hospital and other surrounding hospitals as well as appropriate clinics for teaching[7]. The hospitals and university would be independent institutions, but each would have effective representation on the governing board of the other. This principle was accepted and has continued in operation. The many changes in the health service, especially the introduction of the internal market and the reorganisation of regions in England have, however, put great strain on co-operation between universities, hospitals and other parts of the service.

The Goodenough committee recommended that some medical schools should close[8] and this was done; it suggested that several London schools should move from the centre of the city[9], but many years were to pass before this was accomplished. It proposed with some force that all medical schools become co-educational[10]; only those that admitted 'a reasonable proportion' of women should be eligible for Government funds. The Committee reported that there were large numbers of students in London and Scotland and no medical schools in East Anglia or the south-west of England[11]. Many of the disproportions persist but a clinical school was established in Cambridge in 1976; there is still no medical school south and west of Bristol.

The place of undergraduate education in the health service has been well established in the last 50 years and the introduction of the special increment in funding for undergraduate teaching (SIFT) in 1977 strengthened its place in almost every part of the service. Better defining of SIFT expenditure following the review of 1995[12] allowed funds to be distributed more equitably to teaching and district general hospitals and to general practices according to their teaching contributions. Goodenough would have been pleased.

The pre-registration year

In its 50 meetings, the Committee considered many aspects of its brief. One that found 'enthusiastic support' was the need for a period of supervised, responsible clinical experience after graduation and before full registration[13]. It was noted that before the war about half the graduates, often the least able ones, went straight into practice on completing their course. During the war, many more had completed a house officer post and the Committee recommended that such training be required of all graduates - there should be 'guidance and supervision' throughout. Trainees were to have 'adequate time for thought, for further study, and for the personal investigation of the social and environmental conditions of the patients'; as will be described later, it was a long time before this ideal was even approached, and many would swear that in 50 years of the NHS there was never time for such Elysian arrangements.

The principle of a compulsory pre-registration year was accepted by Government, included in the Medical Act of 1950 and brought into effect on 1 January 1953[14]. Goodenough recommended that two six-months' posts in the year should be in medicine and surgery; posts in obstetrics and gynaecology were rejected by the Committee. The possibility of part of the year being in general practice was also rejected, partly on the grounds that it would be hard to find suitable practitioners who could supervise the trainees[15]. While the opportunity to spend part of the pre-registration period in general practice has existed for some years, it was only in 1997 that the barriers to its wider use were effectively addressed[16]. Government funding for nation-wide introduction of pre-registration training in general practice will commence in 1998.

Postgraduate education

The principles espoused by Goodenough apply equally to undergraduate and to postgraduate medical education (PGME), but the latter has had a more difficult time in gaining acceptance as a full and essential part of the NHS. At the start of the NHS, all junior doctors aspiring to become specialists were considered to be trainees[17]. According to Platt[18] the realities of a new health service had meant that by 1950 only the most senior grade continued to be dedicated to specialist training; training appeared to have become a less essential part of the service. The Platt report was on medical staffing structure but Goodenough would have been astonished to find that while much was said about 'training' and 'experience', the word 'education' was not used.

The senior house officer grade, converted in 1951 from the earlier recommended junior registrar grade, to indicate that not all such juniors were destined to become specialists, was seen in the Platt Report[18] as a resident grade whose members were "normally surely under an obligation to be always at hand day and night, subject to an off-duty rota". Platt found many of the junior staff to be overworked and he made this concession: "though the doctors in the house and registrar grades are there to work as pairs of hands, they are also there as part of the process of preparing themselves for their ultimate careers for which study is still essential".

Perhaps stirred by Platt's report, a meeting took place at Christ Church, Oxford in December 1961 under the chairmanship of Sir George Pickering, that was to be seminal in promoting PGME[19,20]. While Goodenough had seen medical education being built around the teaching centre, the Christ Church conference saw the district hospital as the basic unit for PGME. It recommended the setting up of a postgraduate centre at each training hospital, with library, lecture and seminar facilities, and appointment of a clinical tutor to oversee training in the hospital. A system of regional committees and appointment of a postgraduate dean by the university medical school were also proposed. Pickering may have recalled the recommendation of Goodenough that universities having a medical faculty "should appoint a special committee or board of post-graduate medical studies (and) depute a person to undertake the organisation and general supervision of the post-graduate arrangements ... who might hold the position of dean for postgraduate medical studies"[21].

Postgraduate centres

Postgraduate medical education centres proposed by Pickering were established rapidly, offering a focus of medical education for trainees in the hospitals and general practitioners in the vicinity. Many were funded by local subscription and fund-raising; others came through the generosity of the Nuffield Provincial Hospitals Trust, of which Sir William Goodenough had been chairman. In its annual report for 1964[22] the Nuffield Trust described its enthusiastic assistance for PGME, believing that educational development would "improve hospital and health services in the provinces". Government support for the revival of postgraduate education as a part of the NHS seems to have been limited, however; having provided £250,000 for postgraduate centres and regional and area schemes, the Trust declared its intention to provide no further funds beyond 1967, "to sharpen the focus on the need for ... an official policy (on Government financing)".

In a review of postgraduate education in 1967[23], Revans and McLachlan quoted a paper from the Christ Church conference and declared that "co-ordination between the educational and service authorities hardly exists except in a minor way". At about the same time, a memorandum on postgraduate medical and allied education was issued[24] reminding all hospital authorities of the need to develop facilities for education, but stressing that there would be no further specific allocation of funds for the purpose.

Later reports

In 1968 the Royal Commission chaired by Lord Todd considered PGME to be "haphazard and in many respects unsatisfactory", though big improvements in the development of postgraduate centres were acknowledged[25]. The Todd Report called for greater university involvement and responsibility in the oversight of the pre-registration year, and while looking for greater flexibility in appointments during the year, did not mention the possibility of experience being obtained in general practice. Among many other recommendations, Todd called for the NHS to finance all medical training, including regional postgraduate committees.

The development of postgraduate medical education continued to draw comment and the Merrison Inquiry of 1975 into regulation of the medical profession concluded that "The state of specialist medical education may be likened to the state of undergraduate medical education before control was instituted in the nineteenth century"[26]. If Goodenough's contention was correct, that a strong system of medical education was the essential foundation of a comprehensive health service, then the state of the postgraduate part was a threat to the nation's health.

A development that harks back to Goodenough was the reduction of junior doctors' hours. Even in the darkest days of war and the pressures that were on all staff, Goodenough wrote that trainees must not be overburdened. The Report spoke of "the common practice to make excessive use of the younger men and women in routine work, often to the detriment of their development." Surgical trainees were seen as being greatly overburdened by work, but failing because of lack of time for thought, and poor supervision by seniors, to develop sound judgment.[27] The problems of excessive hours of work were addressed in 1990[28], and Government policy to reduce working hours for trainees at all levels has made fair progress. The problem of supervision of juniors has not been overcome, as evident in a report of the Audit Commission in 1995 where serious deficiencies were reported[29].

The new NHS, 1988

The NHS underwent reorganisation from 1988, and one of the pertinent papers was on PGME[30]. It had echoes of many of the Goodenough principles, asserting again the fundamental importance of education to the service. It restated the need for university medical schools to appoint postgraduate deans, but it gave a new emphasis to the tie between education and the health service, requiring the postgraduate dean to establish standards for education and training and enter agreements with training hospitals that the standards would be met. Even more importantly, the dean was given control of some of the funding of postgraduate education and some leverage by making the meeting of standards a requirement for delivering the funds. In 1993, the lever was lengthened by giving deans 50% of base salaries of trainees, to mark the significance of education and training in the health service[31]. Many have seen advantage in deans having all the funding of base salaries to allow transfer of trainees to sites of optimum education and training. While this has not been accepted by Government, deans now have 100% of funds for pre-registration house officers[32] and public health medicine trainees.

Specialist training revised; the Calman Report

One of the most compelling recommendations of the Goodenough Report was that qualifications and standards of specialist status should be determined by some suitable central machinery and that the primary requisite should be approved postgraduate training and experience of a determined length[33]. Goodenough believed that clinical specialist training required a minimum of 4-5 years after registration, and that during this time the trainee should have adequate time for reading, reflection and research, while being adequately paid, and, as above, being not overloaded with routine work. The Spens Report of 1948[17] expected a graduate of 23-24 years to attain specialist status by the average age of 32. In 1962, Pickering was scathing in his comments on the 10-15 years' training then taken to reach consultant level: "I cannot believe that any responsible body could have so long a period ... the situation has got out of hand".[34]

By 1992, there was Government concern at the duration of specialist training, especially in comparison with training in other European countries, and a review under the chairmanship of the Chief Medical Officer for England, Dr (later Sir) Kenneth Calman reported in 1994[35]. This proposed what Goodenough had recommended, a central machinery and a system for approval of training and experience of determined length. The Report was accepted in full by Government and implemented in stages from December 1995[36]. By early 1997, all 57 specialties were included in the new arrangements: a curriculum set by Colleges; structured programmes of training; progression through the training according to annual assessments; and an end-point of training, the Certificate of Completion of Specialist Training (CCST), administered by a central, statutory authority. There are new recruitment and recording systems administered by postgraduate deans, and new methods of workforce planning. The experience of deans, who combine with medical Royal Colleges to make the system work, is that the new arrangements have greatly improved United Kingdom specialist training. The system continues to evolve, and after 50 years of the NHS this part of medical education meets the expectations of Goodenough and his Committee.

Public support for medical education

Goodenough made much of the importance of public support for medical education and research. "A comprehensive health service must be founded on highly developed and vigorous systems of general and professional education for members of the medical and allied professions, and it must evoke the enthusiastic and intelligent co-operation of the general public"[37]. It may be doubted whether medical education has sought or developed the involvement of the general public, except as subjects for clinical care and study. The current revision of the NHS[38] calls for the participation of the public in all aspects of the service, and after 50 years the ghost of Goodenough would be gratified.

Concluding comment

But what of the leading principle of Goodenough, that medical education is the essential foundation of the health service? The use of the Committee's words 'a healthy nation' in the titles of recent reports *The Health of the Nation*[39] and *Our Healthier Nation*[40] might suggest a link to the Report of 1944. The test, however, is the acceptance after 50 years of the importance of medical education to the NHS and its continuing promotion and development.

The White Paper of 1997 on the new NHS[38] says little about education, and medical education is not mentioned. Goodenough would almost certainly think that there was much still to be done.

References

1. Ministry of Health and Department of Health for Scotland. Compulsory pre-registration house appointments. In: *Report of inter-departmental committee on medical schools*. London: HMSO, 1944; 196-302. Chair: Sir William Goodenough.
2. Beveridge W. *Social insurance and allied services*. London: HMSO, 1942. (Cm. 6404).
3. Editorial. Reform of medical education. *Br Med J* 1944: **2**; 117-118.
4. Ministry of Health and Department of Health for Scotland. *Report of inter-departmental committee on medical schools*. London: HMSO, 1944; 13. Chair: Sir William Goodenough.
5. Ministry of Health and Department of Health for Scotland. *Report of inter-departmental committee on medical schools*. London: HMSO, 1944; 9. Chair: Sir William Goodenough.
6. Rivett G. *From cradle to grave: fifty years of the NHS*. London: King's Fund, 1998; 15.
7. In: *Report of inter-departmental committee on medical schools*. Ministry of Health and Department of Health for Scotland London: HMSO, 1944; 45. Chair: Sir William Goodenough.
8. Ministry of Health and Department of Health for Scotland. *Report of inter-departmental committee on medical schools*. London: HMSO, 1944; 13. Chairman: Sir William Goodenough.
9. Ministry of Health and Department of Health for Scotland. *Report of inter-departmental committee on medical schools*. London: HMSO, 1944; 118. Chair: Sir William Goodenough.
10. Ministry of Health and Department of Health for Scotland. *Report of inter-departmental committee on medical schools*. London: HMSO, 1944; 20. Chair: Sir William Goodenough.
11. Ministry of Health and Department of Health for Scotland. *Report of inter-departmental committee on medical schools*. London: HMSO, 1944; 22. Chair: Sir William Goodenough.
12. Department of Health NHS Executive Advisory Group on SIFT. *SIFT into the future*. London: Department of Health, 1995.
13. In: Ministry of Health and Department of Health for Scotland. Compulsory pre-registration house appointments. *Report of inter-departmental committee on medical schools*. London: HMSO, 1944; 196. Chair: Sir William Goodenough.
14. Department of Health and Social Security. *Royal Commission on medical education 1965-68: report*. London: HMSO, 1968; 42 (Cm. 3569).
15. Ministry of Health and Department of Health for Scotland. *Report of inter-departmental committee on medical schools*. London: HMSO, 1944; 199. Chair: Sir William Goodenough.
16. General Medical Council. *The new doctor*. London: General Medical Council, 1997.
17. Ministry of Health and Department of Health for Scotland. *Report of the inter-departmental committee on the renumeration of consultants and specialists*. London: HMSO, 1948. Chair: Sir W Spens. (Cmd 7470).
18. Ministry of Health and Department of Health for Scotland. *Report of the Joint Working Party on the medical staffing structure in the hospital service*. London: HMSO, 1961; 4-5. Chair: Sir Robert Paltt.
19. Anon. Postgraduate medical education: conference covened by the Nuffield Provincial Hospitals Trust. *Lancet* 1962; **2**: 367-8.
20. Nuffield Provincial Hospital Trust. Conference on postgraduate medical education. *Br Med J* 1962; **1**: 466-467.
21. Ministry of Health and Department of Health for Scotland. *Report of inter-departmental committee on medical schools*. London: HMSO, 1944; 223. Chair: Sir William Goodenough.
22. Nuffield Provincial Hospitals Trust. *Sixth report: a record of the progress of schemes and descriptions of new projects 1961-1964*. London: Nuffield Provincial Hospitals Trust, 1967.
23. Revans J, McLachlan G. *Postgraduate medical education: retrospect and prospect*. London: Nuffield Provicial Hospitals Trust, 1967.
24. Ministry of Health. *Postgraduate medical and allied education*. London: Ministry of Health, 1967 (Health Memorandum: HM(67)33).
25. Department of Health and Social Security. *Royal commission on medical education 1965-68 report*. London: HMSO, 1968; 42 (Cm. 3569).
26. Committee of Inquiry into the Regulation of the Medical Profession. *Report of the committee of inquiry into the regualtion of the medical profession*: London: HMSO, 1975. Chair: Dr AW Merrison. (Cm. 6018).
27. Ministry of Health and Department of Health of Scotland. *Report of inter-departmental committee on medical schools*. London: HMSO, 1944; 213. Chair: Sir William Goodenough.
28. NHS Management Executive. *Hours of work of doctors in training: a new deal*. London: Department of Health, 1991. (Executive Letter: EL(91)82).
29. Audit Commission. *The doctors' tale: the work of hospital doctors in England and Wales*. London: HMSO, 1995.
30. Department of Health NHS Management Executive. *Working for patients: postgraduate and continuing medical and dental education*. London: Deparment of Health, 1991.
31. Department of Health. *Funding of hospital medical and dental training grade posts*. London: Department of Health, 1992 (Executive Letter: EL(92)63).
32. Department of Health. *Review of arrangements for funding postgraduate medical education*. London: Department of Health, 1996. (Executive Letter: EL(96)71).
33. Ministry of Health and Department of Health in Scotland. *Report of the inter-departmental committee on medical schools*. London: HMSO, 1944; 32. Chair: Sir William Goodenough.
34. Pickering G. Postgraduate medical education: the present opportunity and the immediate need. *Br Med J* 1962; **1**: 421-5.
35. Department of Health. *Hospital doctors: training for the future: the report of the Working Group on Specialist Medical Training*. London: Department of Health, 1993. Chair: Dr Kenneth Calman.
36. Department of Health NHS Executive. *A guide to specialist registrar training*. Leeds: Department of Health, 1996.
37. Ministry of Health and Department of Health for Scotland. *Report of inter-departmental committee on medical schools*. London: HMSO, 1944; 9. Chair: Sir William Goodenough.
38. Department of Health. *The new NHS: modern, dependable*. London: Stationery Office, 1997. (Cm. 3807).
39. Department of Health. *The Health of the Nation: a strategy for health in England*. London: HMSO, 1992 (Cm. 1986).
40. Department of Health. *Our Healthier Nation: a contract for health*. London: Stationery Office, 1998 (Cm. 3852).

The National Health Service and the science of evaluation: two anniversaries

John Swales

Director of Research and Development, Department of Health, Room 450 Richmond House, 79 Whitehall, London SW1A 2NS.

Correspondent: Professor John Swales

Health Trends 1998; **30**: 20-2

The National Health Service (NHS) and the first randomised controlled clinical trial came to fruition in the same year[1,2]. It is tempting to refer to this as a happy coincidence but apparent historic coincidences often reflect more fundamental common forces. The demonstration that streptomycin was effective in treating tuberculosis[1] increased dramatically the scope of the new NHS to cure disease and prevent death. Since 1948, the maturation of the NHS has been accompanied by a massive growth both in the volume and the quality of clinical trials. This should surprise no one. Health care requires the information provided by clinical trials, and it could be argued equally persuasively that robust and informative clinical trials require a healthy NHS as a test-bed. I do not propose to discuss the latter relation in this paper.

Patient care and clinical research depend upon each other but service pressures and clinical research are at best uneasy bedfellows. Some recent meticulous analyses from the United States have shown what has been widely felt in this country - that there is, if adequate safeguards are not adopted, a reciprocal relationship between the two[3,4]. This problem is a universal one, although the approach provided by the implementation of the Culyer Taskforce is a novel one adopted in this country. The success of developing a protected research and development levy to fund and support research in the NHS will provide medical historians and perhaps sociologists with a great deal of material. However, rather than discuss the role of the NHS as a test-bed for clinical research I would like to examine the role of evaluative science in the 50-year-old NHS.

Variations in care and evaluation of care

Scientific evaluation in this country did not of course start from scratch in 1948, any more than health care began at that time. Medical interventions have been carried out on frequently unfortunate and ill-advised patients from the earliest days. Such interventions were usually ineffective and often positively harmful. The history of medicine is the replacement of such ineffective means of prevention, diagnosis and treatment with newer, more appropriate and adequately validated technologies. Evaluation therefore fulfils a double role: it is required to establish the validity of what is currently being done and to assess the value of novel interventions which are being proposed to replace existing techniques. If existing ineffective technologies are not abandoned, there will be neither the resources nor the opportunity to replace them with new ones.

The concept that existing treatments might not be effective despite general clinical acceptance is not a particularly new one. Observational studies of variations in care provide some fascinating insights. The pioneer in this field was an Englishman whose work should be more widely recognised. In 1938, J Alison Glover described the rise in the use of tonsillectomy as one of the major phenomena of surgery in England and Wales[5], but one associated with extreme variability (more than twenty-fold in some cases) between adjacent geographical regions. The uneven distribution, he concluded, defied any explanation "save that of variations of medical opinion on the indications for operation". Further, in some areas the incidence of tonsillectomy fell dramatically with loss of local enthusiasm. This fall was attended by no increase in the relevant forms of ill-health for which the operation was carried out. The subsequent discussion of Glover's paper included a telling speculation: "Had a statistician asked that a large control experiment should be arranged by giving and withholding the operation for alternate children and recording their subsequent school medical histories, it would have been met by the usual answer 'if we believe that this treatment is beneficial then it is unfair to withhold it for one half whilst giving it to the other half' ". Such a trial was not done and the annual incidence of tonsillectomy in children waxed and waned over the next few decades.

The NHS had reached the end of its second decade when the existence of unacceptable variations in care again attracted attention and the 'Glover phenomenon' was recognised, although usually not acknowledged as such. Several historic trends contributed to the rapid subsequent growth of evaluative science and the recognition of its role in the NHS (and indeed in other health care systems).

The first of these historic forces was the growth in the success of medical science. This is most obvious, of course, in the development of innovative drugs, but new technologies such as renal dialysis, transplantation, surgical techniques and imaging technology have all contributed. All the evidence points to continuing pressures from the Malthusian growth of science[6]. The pharmaceutical industry, for instance, can now screen millions of compounds in the time required to screen hundreds in the 1970s, and the number of candidate compounds has likewise increased exponentially with the development of combinatorial chemical techniques.

There is every reason to believe that new technologies will continue to offer major challenges and opportunities for all health care systems. The most dramatic of these is probably offered by molecular genetics. This will provide a testing time for the NHS's evaluative procedures. The promise of molecular genetics extends well beyond risk prediction. Indeed, the popular conception that common diseases can be predicted from a sample of cord blood at birth seems a highly unlikely one for the foreseeable future. We cannot readily extrapolate from success in diagnosing monogenetic disorders to success in predicting common multifactorial conditons such as ischaemic heart disease, hypertension, arthritis or asthma. The multiplicity of contributory genes and mutations, and the role of environmental factors, will make prediction a hazardous business. But molecular genetics nevertheless promises different and extremely challenging opportunities in the nearer future. It offers dramatic insight into the biological processes which give rise to disease and therefore provides opportunities for innovative interventions, whether by pharmacological or environmental modification. It provides a potential way to target specific treatments to specific high-risk patients, thereby increasing the efficiency and effectiveness of our interventions. Lastly, we should not forget that other genomes are important to human disease. Sequencing the genomes of the major bacterial pathogens should provide new approaches to such growing problems as antibiotic resistance.

The clinical trial and scientific evaluation

If the picture is one of bewildering growth and complexity, at least we can argue that we are well prepared for this after experience of the advances in science of the last two decades. However, the needs of the health service extend well beyond the assessment of efficacy and scientific validity of claims for new means of diagnosis or prevention or treatment. There are other equally important questions. How are existing services to be modified and new services for health care to be delivered? What are the consequences not simply for the NHS but also for social care and public health? I have purposely laboured the basic message to illustrate the complexity of the questions which have to be addressed.

What does the randomised control trial (RCT) offer us in this situation in its highly developed and sophisticated form, the consequence of 50 years of evolution? We should not underestimate its contribution so far. Treatment offered for common disabling and potentially fatal diseases such as ischaemic heart disease, hypertension, asthma, haematological malignancies, and many other conditions is based upon a robust body of trial-based information.

The use of randomisation was a major step forward but the trial as such has a much longer history. As we have seen, at least one member of Glover's audience regretted that no controlled trial of tonsillectomy had been carried out. But the potential usefulness of the trial method had been recognised long before this. The disturbed genius of Percy Bysshe Shelley, at the beginning of the 19th Century, made impassioned claims for the benefit of a diet of "vegetables and pure water". In the notes to his revolutionary poem *Queen Mab* he defends his position: "On average out of 60 persons 4 will die in 3 years[7]. In April 1914 a statement will be given that 60 persons all having lived more than 3 years on vegetables and pure water are then in perfect health". A (modern) chi-square test shows this difference was indeed significant, although the source of the data would be questioned by a modern trialist. The failure to utilise trial methodology up to more recent years reflects the absence of effective interventions to test. The failure to investigate ineffective methodologies such as, for instance, bleeding and cupping, is an interesting historical reflection on the need to carry out interventions even when no effective intervention was available.

The parallel growth of biomedical and evaluative science during the evolution of the NHS need not surprise us: the pressures of the former generated a need for the latter.

How far can the RCT take us?

Scientific evidence is a necessary but not sufficient contributor to decision-making whether at the policy level or when a professional treats an individual patient. Questions of an individual's value and preferences and of resources also play a necessary role. However, even the application of scientific evidence involves a degree of extrapolation from the trial data to the 'real world'; this applies equally to the patient being treated and to the intervention being used. The Veterans' trial published in 1967 has been enormously influential in guiding treatment of moderate and severe hypertension[8]. Only men were recruited but the methods section of the published report is revealing. In describing the recruitment of patients there is an "additional exclusion" category. Among those excluded were "patients who wished to return to the care of their private physicians, those who for geographical or other reasons would be unable to attend clinic regularly, and patients of dubious reliability such as alcoholics, vagrants and poorly motivated patients". To ensure that only compliant patients were enrolled, potential subjects were given medication which included a fluorescent dye. If the dye was undetectable in a subsequent urine specimen the patient was excluded. Other patient categories have been excluded from trials. No controlled trial of treatment in malignant hypertension or hypertension in children has ever been carried out, nor is it likely that one will ever be undertaken. The development of the clinical trial is not an excuse for abandoning rational judgment in extrapolating from data based upon carefully selected patients to clinical practice.

The same argument applies to the use of interventions in clinical trials. The European Carotid Surgery Trial demonstrated a reduction in disabling or fatal stroke as a result of surgery in patients with a tight carotid stenosis[9]. Postoperative complications in the form of disabling stroke or death were low at 3.7% in a trial which was carried out largely by surgeons in specialist centres. In a community-based study carried out at approximately the same time in Medicare patients this complication rate was 9.8%, a value which would have eliminated the benefits of surgery in the European trial[10]. The 'real world' may not reflect conditions in clinical trials used in guidance for clinicians.

In other situations the randomised control trial is either not feasible or is inappropriate. Public health research sets out to define population interventions which may have a long-term impact upon health. A prospective randomised trial is either unhelpful or prohibitively expensive in this context. This is not to say that efficacy trials have no role. Population strategies for preventing obesity, for instance, may depend upon targeted trials in small groups of subjects for a limited period. The population strategy, however, will be based on much additional relevant evidence which may be largely observational and qualitative rather than prospective and interventional. The argument that we need a prospective trial because one has not been carried out in an important area should be seen for what it is - mechanistic and naive. Clinical trials may also have a more limited role when complex interventions involve several professional disciplines in heterogeneous environments. Social care is a particular example of this. Research into service delivery requires an integration of observational and interventional studies. The value of such work is often not appreciated. Chard *et al* point out that the scientific Western culture is oriented towards quantification[11]; this has yielded enormous returns but the role of qualitative research should not be underestimated, even though qualitative research in medicine is much less frequently cited[11]. In social care it has been much more influential. The Children Act 1989[12], for instance, was strongly influenced by sound research into social work decision-making and child abuse.

The future

The controlled clinical trial and the development of systematic reviews based upon it has been central to progress in the health service over the last 50 years. The two exist in a state of mutual dependence. This will unquestionably continue. Trials of efficacy and pragmatic trials will underpin the incorporation of outputs from new research into health care. Likewise a scientific culture within the health service will help provide an environment in which effective research can be done. However, the complex process of scientific evaluation which is a prerequisite for effective health care requires more than the application of one scientific method. It requires interpretation, integration and extrapolation from knowledge derived from several sources, utilising quite different methods. It is that broad and eclectic approach which will enable the health service to cope with the pressures of scientific advance.

References

1. Streptomycin in Tuberculosis Trials Committee. Streptomycin treatment of pulmonary tuberculosis: a Medical Research Council investigation. *BMJ* 1948; **2**: 769-82.
2. Jadad A R. Rennie D. The randomised controlled trial gets a middle aged checkup. *JAMA* 1998; **279**: 319-20.
3. Moy E, Mazzaschi J, Levin RJ, Blake PH, Griner PF. Relationship between NIH research awards to US medical schools and managed care market penetration. *JAMA* 1997; 278: 217-21.
4. Campbell EG, Weissman JS, Blumenthal D. Relationship between market competition and the activities and attitudes of medical school faculties. *JAMA* 1997; **278**: 222-6.
5. Glover J A. The incidence of tonsillectomy in school children. *Proc R Soc Med* 1938; **31**: 1219-36.
6. Swales J D. *The growth of medical science: the lessons of Malthus.* London: Royal College of Physicians, 1995.
7. Shelley PB. *Queen Mab.* London: PB Shelley, 1813.
8. Veterans Administration Cooperative Study Group on Anti-hypertensive Agents. Effects of treatment on morbidity in hypertension: results in patients with diastolic blood pressures averaging 115 through 129 mmHg. *JAMA* 1967; **202**: 1028-34.
9. European Carotid Surgery Trialists Collaborative Group. MRC European Carotid Surgery Trial; interim results for symptomatic patients with severe (70-90%) or with mild (0-29%) carotid stenosis. *Lancet* 1991; **337**: 1235-43.
10. Winslow CM, Solomon DH, Chassin MR, Kosecoff J, Merrick NJ, Brook RH. The appropriateness of carotid endarterectomy. *N Eng J Med* 1988; **318**: 721-7.
11. Chard JA, Lilford RJ, Court BV. Quantitative medical sociology: What are its crowning achievements? *J R Soc Med* 1997; **90**: 604-9.
12. *The Children Act.* London: HMSO, 1989.

The inspection industry: psychiatry and the National Health Service

Philip Seager

Emeritus Professor of Psychiatry, University of Sheffield (Retired); 9 Blacka Moor Road, Dore, Sheffield S17 3GH.

Correspondent: Professor Seager

Health Trends 1998; **30**: 23-6

On 5th July 1948, I was a fifth-year medical student on obstetric clerking. We attended our ward round to find all the white coated staff, professor to houseman, wearing black armbands - a comment on the formation of the the new National Health Service (NHS). I hope that I felt ashamed at the time (as I did later) but, as students, I expect we found it amusing.

Now we are celebrating (and rightly so), fifty years in action of a great idea. As far as my own specialty of psychiatry is concerned, it brought about truly remarkable changes. We moved from a local authority based 'Cinderella' service to a nationally organised hospital service, with consultants, senior registrars and housemen, just like 'proper' medicine.

To what extent psychiatry has been integrated into the medical profession is too broad a question to answer here. This article looks at aspects of the care of the mentally disordered, the way in which they have been mistreated and abused over the centuries and what has happened during the days of the NHS to change things.

Past abuses
It is no new problem that is being discussed. The 1403 Chancery Roll is the report of the Commission of Enquiry sent to Bethlem Hospital, specifically to investigate the scandals which had been taking place there - not confined, however, to insane patients[1]. The Privy Council set up another Commission of Enquiry to investigate malpractices at Bethlem in 1632-33.

It is probable that much of the early mistreatment related to the view that lunatics and defectives were not normal human beings and did not merit the care that might be otherwise have been given. Laws concerning vagrancy covered a wide range of wanderers, varying in composition according to the views of the day. They came to include lunatics in 1714 but provided only for detention and not for treatment, which came later, in 1744[2].

Parry-Jones[2] quotes observations describing abuse in private madhouses which would turn any person insane. He notes that, while there is little doubt that incarceration in such places was used to obtain access to money and possessions of well-to-do individuals, the effect of caring for violent abusive patients by largely ignorant, untrained attendants, supervised by inadequately trained (and sometimes ignorant) medical staff resulted in a circular situation, which has still been noted on occasions.

Legal issues
Jones[3] outlines the battle between the legalistic approach of the law-makers and the therapeutic attitude of the physicians towards the most effective management of psychiatric patients. The pendulum has swung from one to the other, with the Lunacy Act 1890[4] largely devoted to rigid care authorised by a magistrate and the Mental Treatment Act 1930[5] introducing the concept of voluntary treatment for at least a proportion of patients. It resulted in the acceptance of such terms as 'doctor, nurse, hospital' in the field of psychiatry.

The Royal Commission[6] led to the broad minded (medically speaking) Mental Health Act[7] in which the great majority of patients were assumed to have informal status. They were treated with compulsion, only in the same way as a person found unconscious by the roadside would be treated and operated on to relieve immediate crisis. It was the doctor who made the decisions about whether and what kind of treatment was required.

The power this was seen to give the psychiatrists resulted in outcries led largely by Larry Gostin[8], at that time Legal Adviser to the mental health charity Mind, and influential in the design of proposals for a new Mental Health Act by the then Labour Government. Political considerations of quite another kind led to a change of administration and the eventual Mental Health Act 1983[9], while much more caring for the rights of the patient, still allowed medical decision in the treatment of those who were mentally ill.

The Board of Control, a supervisory body dating from the Lunacy Act[4] had been disbanded in 1959; the new Act introduced the Mental Health Act Commission, one of whose tasks was to compile a code of practice for use in psychiatric management. First drafts produced unwieldy textbooks of parapsychiatry, composed by a committee of 90 members including nurses, lawyers, teachers, doctors, administrators and even a few psychiatrists. Fortunately this was abandoned and subsequent Codes of Practice have produced more realistic ideas of relevant guidance.

Recent reports of abuse
Reference has already been made to vivid descriptions of the care, or lack of care found in earlier centuries. But these problems are evidently not confined to times gone by. In 1957, The Plea for the Silent[10], edited by two Members of Parliament, Dr Donald Johnson and Mr Norman Dodds, exposed abuses in mental hospitals. It was not till the 1960s that one began to hear

of systematic reporting of specific abuse of vulnerable individuals, whether elderly[11], mentally ill or mentally handicapped[12].

Robb[11] set out the evidence of six nurses and two social workers concerning demeaning, and often vicious behaviour by staff towards elderly patients, ostensibly being cared for in a range of wards for the elderly in psychiatric and geriatric hospitals in England. Names of staff, patients and hospitals were disguised to prevent identification and scapegoating, but are held by the publishers as affidavits and vouched for by the author.

Martin[12] reviewed eight inquiries in abuses at mental illness hospitals, one at a Special Hospital and four at mental handicap hospitals, during the period 1969 to 1980. He briefly mentions a further three 'local' inquiries, carried out by members of the health auhority and individual prosecutions of staff for serious breaches of their duty of care. He also refers to publication of reports in national newspapers after visits by the National Development Team and the Health Advisory Service.

NHS Trusts should have arrangements in place to investigate and, where necessary, report to the relevant health authority serious incidents. More recently, health authorities have been required to commission an independent inquiry if a homicide is committed by a person with mental illness. These reports are usually published and often receive media attention. It is interesting to speculate what makes a particular story national news, compared with others which receive only little or no mention in the local press and radio. Often, it is a particularly bizarre or frightening murder, especially of a complete stranger, but it is probably more likely that it depends on the drive and enthusiasm of a local individual, or even the dearth of other exciting news at that moment.

The Confidential Inquiry into Homicides and Suicides by Mentally Ill People[13] indicates the relative rarity of homicide by psychiatric patients, approximately 20% of the 400-500 homicides annually. Where it occurs, family members are almost always the victim, with members of staff on five occasions and in three, total strangers. Suicide is considerably more common with highly variable antecedents, even in those under continuing or recent psychiatric care. Key problems identified by the Inquiry included failure of communication between professionals, lack of clarity concerning care plans, lack of time for face-to-face contact, need for additional staff training, poor compliance with treatment and insufficient use of legal powers to supervise at-risk patients.

One would expect that the effect of all these inquiries and consequent publicity would have some effect on the incidence of damaging behaviour to vulnerable people kept in care because they are not able to exist on their own. Sadly, this does not appear to be the case, and indeed the many organisations which have come into being because of this spate of inquiries seem equally limited in their effects.

The inspection industry
I would like to examine the range of visitors assessing the scope of care and treatment at a typical psychiatric service, whether mental hospital, general hospital unit or other form of care.

The first responsibility lies with those who manage the unit. Senior managers should visit all the facilities in their charge, looking at the buildings and the environment, and most importantly, giving all staff, both day and night, the opportunity to outline problems and difficulties and exchange ideas about improvement of patient care. In addition, there is need for a system of confidential access to someone who can listen to doubts and anxieties and act on information without the person feeling at risk of blame or criticism, even if the the complaint is unwarranted. The right to report breaches of rules was recognised and is now mandatory for doctors registered with the General Medical Council.

The authority has varied in the degree to which it is supervised by its senior authority, depending on the particular organisation in play at the time. Nevertheless, since public money is at stake, there is always some higher supervisory power, whether at regional, Department of Health, or Audit Commission level. Essentially, their role is comparative, ensuring that the standards availabe locally are those shared by the service as a whole. It also offers the opportunity of passing round ideas and methods of modifying and improving specific methods of management and care.

In addition to these statutory controls, most professional organisations take more than a passing interest in the services in which their staff carry out their duties. This is true of trade unions and professional organisations alike. It is particularly important to those bodies responsible for the education and training for entrants to their profession. As a result, visitors from the appropriate national Nursing Board, the local College of Nursing, the Royal Colleges of Psychiatry, General Practice, Medicine, Nursing and other professionals organisations in occupational therapy, social work, pharmacy, art therapy all look not only at the teaching facilities and the details of implementation of the curriculum, but also at the environment in which their students are working and the attitudes of the senior staff who should be models of good practice.

But there is more. Arising out of the Ely enquiry by Geoffrey Howe in 1969[14], Richard Crossman, the Minister of Health set up the NHS Hospital Advisory Service, "one of the two best things I ever did". It began by visiting all hospital services for the elderly, the mentally ill and mentally handicapped in England and Wales and reporting on each visit directly to the Minister of Health. Soon after it started, there had been a change of Government and Sir Keith Joseph, the new Minister, took a personal interest in the reports which came to his desk.

Later changes which took place included separating off mental handicap services to the supervision of the National Development Team, forming a joint partnership with the Social Services Inspectorate and publishing the hitherto confidential reports. It extended its remit to community as well as hospital services and was renamed the Health Advisory Service.

Multiprofessional teams of five or six spent periods of up to three weeks in health districts, meeting staff, patients, relatives and general practitioners. They gave a report to the staff at the end of the visit and a written report was submitted to the Minister and back to the District some weeks later.

The Social Services Inspectorate, in addition to its role with the HAS, included community services for the mentally ill in its local authority visits but eschewed the advantage of using mental health professionals. But within local authority services themselves, Approved Social Workers had the opportunity to fulfil their advice to provide the least restrictive type of treatment environment when they made an application for compulsory admission. They could have questionned the absence of a range of options rather than just accepting what was available. All too often, however, they were only too aware of the dearth of alternative non-hospital accommodation.

In 1989, the Department of Health established a Clinical Standards Advisory Group under the Chairmanship of Professor John Richmond. This was intended to apply standards of high quality clinical care as models for the acute services. Due to the enthusiasm of the then President of the Royal College of Psychiatrists, they took on the task in relation to services for patients suffering from schizophrenia; they found them sadly lacking in a number of important aspects.

The Mental Health Act Commission, set up by statute, pursued its task of ensuring that patients detained under the Mental Health Act 1983[9], were receiving appropriate care and treatment and all patients were able to seek interviews with them if they felt aggrieved. Members of the Commission paid regular visits to hospitals in rotation and monthly visits to the Special Hospitals where the scope for difficulties was seen to be greater. These regular visits to Ashworth Hospital did not prevent a number of major difficulties at that hospital[15].

Another opportunity of review of patients lies with the Mental Health Review Tribunals. Patients detained under sections of the Mental Health Act 1983[9] have the right to apply for review of their detention at prescribed intervals. If they do not avail themselves of this opportunity, the hospital must refer them for assessment. The tribunal, composed of a lawyer, psychiatrist and 'lay' person, usually with social work or similar experience, all unconnected with the hospital, review reports and hear comments from the Responsible Medical Officer, social worker, usually the named nurse, often a family member and the patient and his or her legal representative. They make a decision as to whether the compulsory order is allowed to stand or should be rescinded.

Most recently, in the Mental Health Act for England and Wales, 1983, managers have been given responsibility for receiving and scrutinising documents in relation to detention of each patient, though this may be delegated to responsible officers. More important is their responsibility for ensuring that good practice is observed and that services are adequate for the demands made on them. They also have the role of hearing appeals from those detained and reviewing renewals of detention. This has proved contentious as three managers have the statutory power after scrutiny of reports from the Responsible Medical Officer and other professional staff and interviewing the patient to decide to revoke detention. This has led to some professional disquiet and a working group of members of the Mental Health Act Commission, the Royal College of Psychiatrists and the National Association of Hospitals and Trusts suggested this policy should be changed. However, this could only be brought about by ammending the 1983 Act[9] so any such change would have to await a broader consideration of the whole Act. Some regard this role as a duplication of the work of the Mental Health Review Tribunals which are charged with an independent review function.

Because patients were felt to have little or no opportunity of accessing the local health services, Community Health Councils were established in each authority by the new administrative machinery in 1973. These Councils, intended to represent the average person, tended to be filled by people with various specialist axes to grind. Their strength depended largely on their paid secretary. While they had the right of access to health authority minutes, attended their meetings and had a say before the closure of any local hospital, opinions about their merits varied widely. An individual with a health grievance could get the ear of a campaigning secretary, who would act as his advocate and obtain a hearing, probably a letter of apology and some constructive action to rectify the problem. They are also prepared to press for improvement in limited resources.

One might expect this extensive list of visitors to the psychiatric and geriatric services, carried out by experienced knowledgeable professionals of goodwill and concern to improve the quality of the services under review. But still the tragedies occur, the inquiries continue and a collection of reports gathers dust somewhere within the depths of numerous authority archives. These inquiries are not without cost - not only in financial terms, though they do provide an income for retired professionals - but also in the organisation and planning of appointments, interviews with staff who must be released from their main duties, and the stress caused to patients and their families, to staff, who rightly or wrongly feel they are being accused of malfeasance, and to the general feeling of unease when a group of inquirers descend on a unit, asking strange, often incomprehensible questions.

Conclusions

It is important to examine the situation to try and identify the reasons for the breakdown in the normal process of compassion and care for disabled individuals.

The onus is still on the professional to understand and sympathise with people who are frightened or shocked by their recent experience, see themselves in a strange environment where they feel at a disadvantage, and respond by aggression, at first minor, but rapidly escalating if not handled properly. This is even more so if the person suffers from other disadvantages, whether of sex, race, language or pre-existing mental illness.

Can there be a problem with our own staff? They are ostensibly well trained, well paid so that they can respond to all the demands made on them, with time for face to face discussions with patients and relatives, and opportunities for specialist training and advice. One can only assume that many of the problems which we see at the moment rise from the changes which are happening in the pace and the place of psychiatric care.

Selection of staff, adequacy of numbers and opportunities for continuing training and education are the essential prerequisites of a good workforce. Moves from the shelter of large confined units to the much more stressful services provided in small units with limited access to advice and help lead to personal difficulties which are then compounded by a lowering of morale which discourages new entrants.

This is not to suggest that the changes which have taken, and are taking place are inappropriate or unsuitable. On the contrary, help is best given in small packets, perhaps in, or near the individual's home, or at least in a home-like atmosphere. But some of the package may lack the necessary feeling of expertise and confidence in the professional. Asking 'What would you like me to do?' is not the same as ensuring that the patient understands what the treatment plan is and is prepared to participate because it has all been made clear.

We have to get the right balance between being friendly and welcoming, and being relaxed and unprofessional so that the patient has no confidence that anyone knows what is necessary to be done. We have to recognise that we are in a position of power, and this is largely because the patient needs to have some sense of support and well being as part of the therapeutic environment in which treatment is being offered.

It is a sad fact that there will always be crises, disasters and cruelty shown by a few to the vulnerable who need help and suport. The Royal College of Psychiatrists hold in its Library, an extensive list of Inquiries held over the past three decades· The Zito Foundation has rapidly issued two editions of its report on Inquiries[16], indicating their proliferation. It is arguable whether inspection is the way to resolve such problems. In the end it comes down to the professional awareness and confidence of staff who recognise malpractice and take active appropriate steps to resolve it before damage is done. A trite council of perfection, maybe, but one which is necessary to achieve a better record over the next 50 years of NHS psychiatry.

References

1. Allderidge. [Archivist & Curator, Bethlem Royal Hospital & Museum]. Personal communication. S.l.: Patricia Allderidge, s.d.
2. Parry-Jones WL. *The trade in lunacy: a study of private madhouses in England in the eighteenth and nineteenth centuries*. London: Routledge & Kegan Paul, 1971.
3. Jones. *Law and mental health: sticks or carrots?* In: Berrios German E, Freeman, eds. *150 Years of British psychiatry 1841-1991*. London: Gaskell, 1991; 89-102.
4. *The Lunacy Act*. London: HMSO, 1890.
5. *The Mental Treatment Act*. London: HMSO, 1930.
6. Royal Commission on the Law Relating to Mental Illness and Mental Deficiency. Report. London: HMSO, 1957 (Cm. 169).
7. *The Mental Health Act*. London: HMSO, 1959.
8. Gostin LO. *A human condition*. London: MIND, 1976.
9. *The Mental Health Act*. London: HMSO, 1983.
10. Johnson D McI, Dodds N. *The plea for the silent*. London: Johnson, 1957.
11. Robb. *Sans everything: a case to answer*. London: Nelson, 1967.
12. Martin JP. *Hospitals in trouble*. Oxford: Blackwell, 1984.
13. Steering Committee of the Confidential Inquiry into Homicides and Suicides by Mentally Ill People. *Report of the confidential inquiry into homicides and suicides by mentally ill people*. London: Royal College of Psychiatrists, 1996.
14. Crossman R. *The diaries of a cabinet minister*. London: Cape Hamilton, 1977. (Vol. 3).
15. Committee of Inquiry into Complaints About Ashworth Hospital. *Report of the committee of inquiry into complaints about Ashworth Hospital*. London: HMSO, 1992.
16. Sheppard D. *Learning the lessons*. 2nd ed. London: Zito Trust, 1996.

Guidelines for authors

If you submit a paper to *Health Trends*, you **must** supply:

- the original paper plus four copies;

- a covering letter signed by all the authors;

- the questionnaire used in the research or study (if applicable); *and*

- proof that when research on patients/clients or their records is reported, LREC approval was secured.

If these criteria are not fully met, the paper will be returned without consideration.

Submission of papers:

Topics for inclusion in *Health Trends* should be related to medical aspects of National Health Service practice, management, planning, implementation and evaluation. Original contributions from a variety of disciplines are welcome and must be submitted exclusively to *Health Trends*. The readership is general and international; authors should avoid 'jargon' terms or concepts used by a particular specialty. Papers are accepted for publication on their scientific originality and general interest, and on the understanding that they will be subjected to editorial revision. Papers and accompanying material will not be returned to authors unless specifically requested.

The original paper and four copies accompanied by a covering letter containing the signature of all co-authors should be submitted to the Editor at the address shown on the inside front cover of the Journal. If a research questionnaire was used in the study, it should be enclosed. All papers will be acknowledged, and authors will be notified of a paper's accceptance or rejection once the review process is complete. A reference number will be given for enquiries and *must* be quoted in any communications with the Medical Editorial Unit. *Papers based on research involving patients/clients or their records, must indicate in the text that the research had the prior approval of the appropriate ethics committee; proof of this is also required*[1].

Authorship:

Persons should qualify to be designated as authors only if they have contributed substantially to: the design of the study; analysis of the data; *and* drafting or critically revising the article. Acquisition of funding alone for the research should not justify authorship. The order of authorship may be altered by the Editor to suit journal style or format.

Referees:

Papers accepted for consideration will be reviewed independently by a panel of referees. The Editor retains ultimate responsiblity for the refereeing process.

Presentation of papers:

Authors should examine a copy of *Health Trends* for examples of Journal style, expression and lay-out. Normally, papers should not exceed 2,000 words, or contain more than six tables. The paper should be typed in double spacing, on one side only of A4 paper. Each author should indicate his/her professional discipline and current appointment. Authors should keep at least one copy of their paper for reference. The paper should indicate the person to whom proofs and inquiries are to be sent, their full address (including postal code), a telephone and FAX number, and the name of a co-author (if applicable) who can provide information to the Editorial Unit when the correspondent is unavailable.

Headings:

Papers should follow the usual convention, ie title page; summary; introduction; method; results; discussion; acknowledgements; references; tables and figures.

Data and terminology:

All quantitative measurements should be in terms of the International System of Units (SI), but blood pressure should continue to be expressed in mm Hg. All drugs and other compounds should be referred to by their accepted generic names, and not by their proprietary names, unless it is essential for clarification purposes. Statistical methods should be defined, and any not in common use should be described in detail or supported by references. Where percentages are given within the text and tables, the actual number of patients/clients on which these are based should also be provided.

Tables:

Tables accompanying papers should be identified by Arabic numerals, typed in double spacing on separate sheets of paper (ie, not incorporated within written text). Authors should indicate an appropriate position within the text for tables and/or figures. The title of the table should be brief, but the contents should contain a clear and complete explanation of what the data represent. Footnotes should be included only where necessary, to clarify the data and to give a fuller descripton of compact headings. Data contained in the tables should supplement, not duplicate, information in the written text.

Figures and graphs:

Figures and graphs should leave the reader in no doubt about the kind of objects, events, people or measurements represented; the units used; the geographical coverage; the time period covered; the scale of measurements; the source(s) of the data; and how to interpret the chart. Any material previously published, or unpublished, should be accompanied by the wrtten consent of the copyright holder; full acknowledgement and references must be given. Graphs should be presented as clear line drawings on white paper or graph paper. Data used to determine value 'points' indicated *must* accompany all graphs.

References:

The accuracy and completeness of references are important, *and are the authors' responsibility*. A maximum of 20 key references per paper should be numbered consecutively in the order in which they appear in the text. At the end of the paper, a full list of references should be presented in Vancouver style[2]; references must not be in the form of footnotes in the text.

Acknowledgements:

Only those who have made substantial contribution to the study and/or preparation of the paper should be acknowledged. The sources of grants, equipment and drugs should be included. Authors should obtain permission from people acknowledged by them, as readers may infer their endorsement of the data and conclusion published.

Correspondence:

Letters must *only* relate directly to recently published articles, and must be limited to a maximum of 450 words. Letters may also be submitted for reviewers' comments. The Editor reserves the right to edit all correspondence, and to decide if, and when, correspondence should be published. Letters must be signed by all the authors.

Publication process:

An edited version of the paper will be sent to authors for their comments/approval prior to publication. The page-proofs will then be sent by FAX (or post) to the corresponding author, who is responsible for checking the type-setting accuracy thoroughly and giving written consent for publication. Alterations to the text are best avoided at this stage, and in general only essential updating amendments will be accepted.

References

[1] Department of Health. *Local Research Ethics Committee*s. Heywood (Lancashire): Department of Health, 1991 (Health Service Guidelines: HSG(9I)5).

[2] International Committee of Medical Journal Editors. Uniform requirements for manuscripts submitted to biomedical journals. *JAMA* 1993; **269**: 2282-6.

Further reading

[1] Guidelines for writing papers. *BMJ* 1989; **298**: 40-42.

Indexing/Abstract Service

Health Trends is indexed by the Hospital Literature Index, American Hospital Association Resource Center, 840 North Lake Shore Drive, Chicago, IL 60611. It is also indexed in the Health Planning and Administration File and the HEALTH database on the MEDLARS system at the US National Library of Medicine, Bethesda, Maryland, USA. The Journal is indexed and abstracted by Excerpta Medica, Elsevier Science Publishers B.V., PO Box 2227, 10000 CE Amsterdam, The Netherlands.

Notification of change of address

When notifying a change of address, please quote any reference number shown on the label used to send *Health Trends* to you.

Doctors in contract with the NHS and receiving free copies should notify The Medical Mailing Company, PO Box 60, Derby Road, Loughborough, Leicestershire LE11 0WP.
Freephone Medical Mailing 0800 626387.

Other recipients of free copies should notify the Medical Editorial Unit in writing.

Subscribers should write to Subscriptions Department, The Stationery Office Publications Centre, 51 Nine Elms Lane, London SW8 5DR.

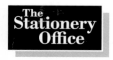

Published by The Stationery Office and available from:

The Publications Centre
(mail, telephone and fax orders only)
PO Box 276, London SW8 5DT
General enquiries 0171 873 0011
Telephone orders 0171 873 9090
Fax orders 0171 873 8200

The Stationery Office Bookshops
123 Kingsway, London WC2B 6PQ
0171 242 6393 Fax 0171 242 6394
68–69 Bull Street, Birmingham B4 6AD
0121 236 9696 Fax 0121 236 9699
33 Wine Street, Bristol BS1 2BQ
0117 9264306 Fax 0117 9294515
9–21 Princess Street, Manchester M60 8AS
0161 834 7201 Fax 0161 833 0634
16 Arthur Street, Belfast BT1 4GD
01232 238451 Fax 01232 235401
The Stationery Office Oriel Bookshop
The Friary, Cardiff CF1 4AA
01222 395548 Fax 01222 384347
71 Lothian Road, Edinburgh EH3 9AZ
0131 228 4181 Fax 0131 622 7017

The Stationery Office's Accredited Agents
(see Yellow Pages)

and through good booksellers

£7.50
Annual Subscription £28.00

ISBN 0-11-781561-6

9 780117 815612 >